MIND ON FIRE

A Wild Trip Through a Bipolar Life

NINO BRODEUR

Imprint

© 2022 Nino Brodeur
e-mail: mind.on.fire.nino.brodeur@gmail.com
Internet: http://www.mind-on-fire.us
Covergestaltung: Lars Hütz - 4h-digital.de
Lektorat, Korrektorat: Julia Schoch,
Fotos: Thomas Hartmann, http://www.h2creativ.de
Production and publishing: IngramSpark

ISBN Paperback: 979-8-218-01339-4

Photos, videos, comments and everything about
this book are available on:

www.mind-on-fire.us

Facebook: Mind-on-Fire

facebook.com/Cosmokraut72

Instagram: mind.on.fire.nino.brodeur

To all people who, like me, have psychological problems
and sometimes don't know what to do. To my family,
who loves and supports me anyway. And a greeting
to every rocker who does his own thing.

Table of Contents

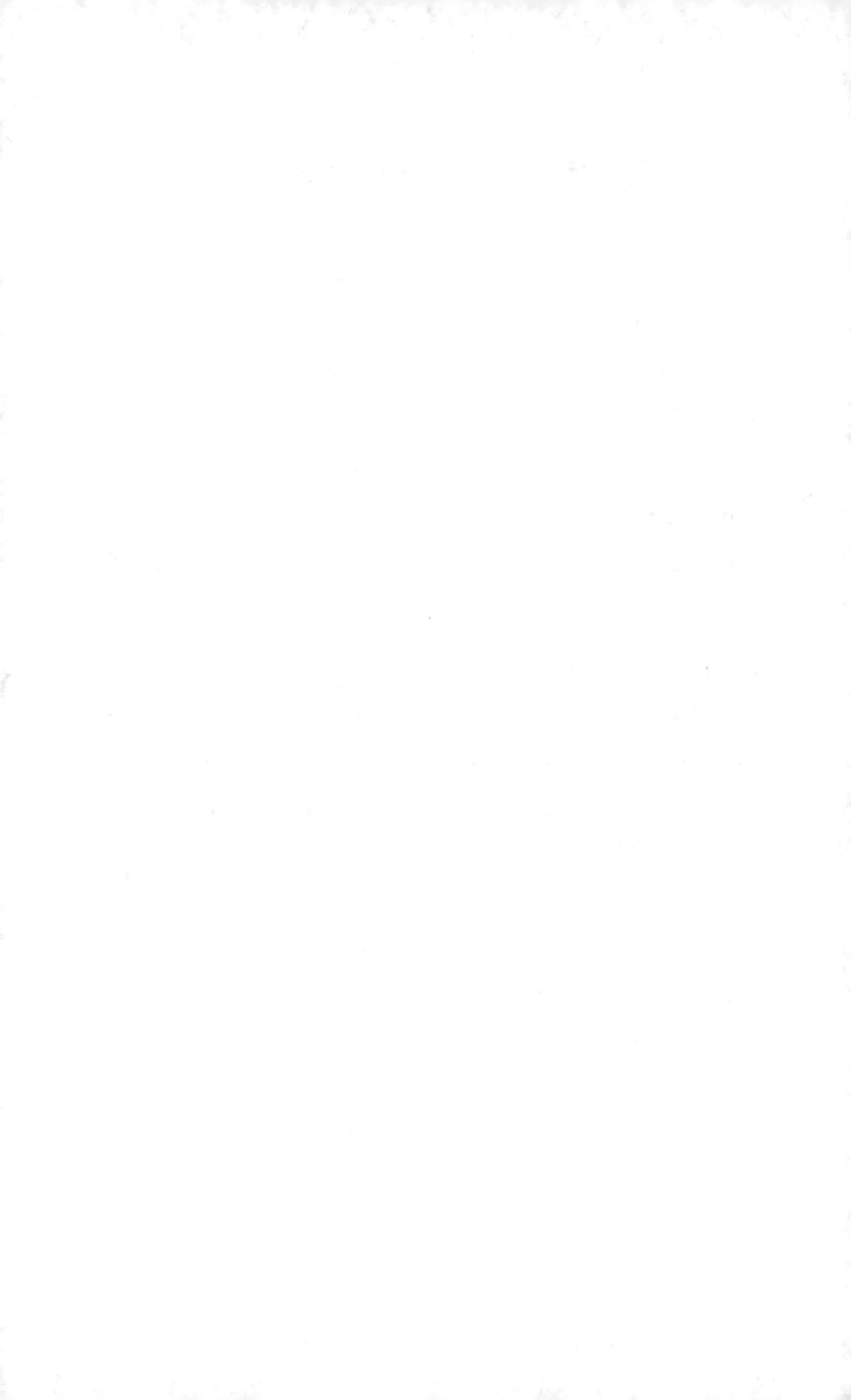

Introduction

7:00 a.m., clinic/psychiatric ward

»Mr. Brodeur ... Mr. Brodeur!!!«
»What? What's going on?«
»We would like to activate you.«
»You want to what?«
»Activate you.«

Once again landed in the loony bin - sad routine. They know me there and – pee on the wall - I know them.

I feel empty, numb, and can't wait to read the soft-flushed, bloated, drug-soaked faces as the inmates butter their rolls in slow motion in the morning. And then the silent, crowded and slow elevator on the way down for a cigarette ... yes, that's great cinema.

My good friend Ralf died two weeks ago. It was probably the heart. So young. I lost control again and my brain got really fucked again.

I am bipolar or also manic-depressive.

<u>Mania:</u> My head is so flooded with feelings of happiness and absurd strength that I lie down on Mainstreet at night and am sure that no car can harm me. My mind is running incredibly fast. All the other people around me don't seem to understand anything. A veritable fireworks display takes place in my head. I don't notice that I have already far exceeded the limit. The collapse comes, my brain goes haywire, I fight it aggressively and then desperate tears flow.

Depression: Head and body are completely exhausted after the mania. I spend days or even weeks staying in bed, unable to accomplish anything. I feel only deep sadness, totally exhausted. I lie there watching all the crap on TV. I manage to go to the bathroom, but that's about it. I cry uncontrollably sometimes and sleep easily 16 hours a day. It's like black tar is pouring over my brain. I am not living. The depression is sucking the life out of me. Depression is when you can no longer feel things you normally love.

These extreme states can change very quickly, but can also last for weeks and months. They are called type 1 and type 2. The stronger and longer the mania is, the more violent and longer the depression follows.

Also, in mania, drugs that promote excess are usually a part of the disease. Artists and manic-depressive people both tend to have ecstatic moments, grand gestures, and rampant concepts. Manic persuasion of others is extremely strong.

My name is Nino, I came into this world in 1972 and my favorite movie is *Leolo*.

Before you read this book, I must mention that it is written somewhat erratically. That's also part of the clinical picture. I flip back and forth between thoughts pretty quickly. That said, I do my best to make the book entertaining, humorous, but also serious.

My goals:

1. I want tell my story and hope that those people affected by the disease will find themselves in it.
2. I want to make it easier for friends, and especially family members, to understand this disease. Communication is very important and I believe that it is possible to shape the future together.

On the second point, I would like to say that the environment is usually helpless. It is not a broken arm. It happens in the brain and it is difficult to help. You can recognize Depression by the fact that you can no longer feel things that you actually love.

Therapies and medications can do their part in recovery. However, to be honest, after all this time I realize that I basically have to live with it forever. All attempts to cure my dilemma have failed miserably to date. It's a constant struggle and it's very difficult to persevere. I am dead serious about that. I have experienced a lot of love in my life and that is what I believe in, that is why I am still here.

I ask you not to look for answers to your psychological problems in the book. I am not a doctor or a pharmacist. I am describing how it happened to me. It is my life story, nothing more, nothing less. Manic-depressive illness does not go away, it is always there. But it is important that you, your family and your friends learn to deal with it. Then it will not be so difficult for you to live your life.

A slight negativity is also noticeable. I am not writing to draw attention to beautiful things. That time heals all wounds is not true. A scar tissue forms around the pain and every now and then it shimmers through.

I would love to please everyone all the time, but that is not possible in this book. I can't accommodate the demands of everyone involved, name changes will have to suffice. Everything I tell happened exactly like that. I describe the course of my life from my point of view, of course, and make assumptions about the minds of other people.

Sex, drugs and rock 'n' roll are components of this book. It may not be right for squeamish readers.

**»You're asking me what to do? Live wild and dangerous, Arthur.«
Nothing is true, everything is allowed.**

At the moment, I'm still in psychotherapy, and the health insurance company has approved another year. Sometimes I have the feeling that my therapist proceeds according to a timed pattern, but there are also aha-effects that help me further. Every once in a while, her intent is very obvious. She asks questions and I know exactly what that's aimed at. It's okay, she's basically examining me and that's her craft. All in all, I'm glad because there have been about five therapists before her over the years. It is very important that the chemistry between the patient and the therapist is right, otherwise therapy is of no use at all.

I was born in Berlin and my favorite bands are The Doors and Element of Crime.

Not being able to allow closeness was and still is a big problem, I think many people feel this way. In my relationships, this was always an elementary disruptive factor. An unhappy state, to love and not be able to show it or live it out - at least not in the way I want to. I have hurt many women without wanting to. The search for security and the seething desire to show who I really am - I never succeeded. I experienced the love of my girlfriends and could not give back enough. My ex-wife always accused me of living in the past.

I firmly believe that the past, the now and the future belong together and should be perceived as a whole.

Nothing gets on my nerves more than people who force themselves to always see everything positively. Nobody can stand that in the long run. Life offers the full range of emotions to live out. Most of the time, the 'pseudo-positives' have been hurt badly in the past. That's tragic, but it's not an answer. The spiritual bubble is associated with egomania. Towards other people they are usually inconsiderate and they behave in a derogatory and arrogant way. Living for the moment, okay, but a mayfly will never be able to understand anything historical or intellectually conscious. I mention this because I have had intense experience with it. It is certainly not true in general. Diversity is everything and of course every person should become and be happy in her or his own way.

However, I fully agree with the attitude of being grateful for everything. A good view of things.

It is wonderful to look at a person and be able to grasp the whole being. I guess that's what you call empathy. I always feel a tingling sensation, I just smile a bit strangely and am happy. In mania, however, this ability contributes to the fact that even more emotions and information affect me unintentionally.

What is equally important is that the bipolar has feelings of guilt. I often feel like a burden to my family, powerless to change anything. Friends usually don't know where to place me.

Family

My family is always there for me and supports me. That helps me get through difficult crises. I love my family very much and am grateful for my friends. Experiencing myself in a normal state is unfortunately rare. In the meantime, I hardly know what that is.

My sister Luisa is three years younger than me and a doctor by profession. She has a similarly sensitive psyche as I do. In elementary school, she had a class teacher with whom she absolutely couldn't get along. I don't know what exactly happened, but she suddenly became hard of hearing. All kinds of things were examined and my parents feared that something was wrong in the brain. It was the psyche. After she changed schools, her hearing also came right back. Damn powerful organ, that psyche.

It's hard for me to write about my mother. She always takes everything so much to heart. She wants to let bygones be bygones. When I look at old pictures of my parents, I can only guess how much they used to love and live. From my mother I have inherited the world-weariness. She gave me her strong emotionality and many character traits come from my father. I am so fifty-fifty.

There were some incidents in my mother's extended family circle: Depression, addiction, suicide. So I conclude that there is a genetic pre-programming in me.

My sister, on the other hand, has used recessive genes and she is aware of that. She had a picture of Grandma on her desk from a young age, she felt the connection to her. Luisa is beautiful and aloof, introverted. She rarely speaks on an emotional level. Still, her and I are kindred spirits. Anyone who has siblings knows this: a situation, a moment. You look at each other and start laughing, words are not necessary.

At one point in her life she knew what she wanted and fought for it. I always wanted to have kids, she did. I envy her for that. Well, two women that I know of were pregnant by me, one from Norway and one from Bremen. I haven't heard from them and it's been a long time ago.

I hope to be a good uncle to my sister's two boys. But now let's go ...

Childhood

I was wrapped in a blanket. I heard a woman's voice.

»Ohhh, what's that? A package ... for me? What might be in it?«
Then the blanket opened and I was told to answer, »Me.«
»Ohhhh, it's Nino.« the woman's voice rejoiced.

I was just five years old and already in therapy. I didn't really like the world and stuttered. I think my father put that in the gene pool. He used to have problems with it, too. The therapist tried to build up my self-confidence. Even as a little boy, I had very little self-confidence. I watched other kids play and lived in my own world. That hasn't changed to this day; I still live in my own world and observe, that's okay. With time I got better and got rid of my stutter too.

Around the same time I started playing sports. I played mainly field hockey and tennis, and in the winter I learned to ski. Until I was 14, I was active in sports for many hours every day. We were always a sports family and half of our time was spent in a tennis and field hockey club. This is still the case. My father's loyalty to the club was not always met with approval on my mother's side. He was rarely at home, either working in other countries or enjoying life at the sports club. For myself, sports helped me develop good social behavior. Tennis is probably more of an ego game - I don't know how many rackets I smashed - but fortunately field hockey is a team sport and prevented worse.

I remember that in the beginning we used to get coal briquettes from the cellar for heating when I was a child. My mother's favorite smell was 'cellar'. Our TV had no remote control and we received a whole five channels. I was a *Superman* fan. I was often caught reading comics in stores without buying them. My buddy Henry and I loved *YPS* magazines. Every time we had sleepovers together, we would tinker with the *YPS* gimmicks. We were especially fond of the glowing green dinosaur skeletons. The Mexican jumping beans weren't bad either, and of course we liked everything that had to do with espionage and detectives - that's just the way it is with boys.

I wasn't much of a reader as a kid, my extracurricular reading is easy to list: *The Little Vampire*, *The Little Ghost*, *Sherlock Holmes* and *The Neverending Story*.

China I

My father received an offer from his company to build a steel mill in China. It would be worthwhile, he agreed. What an adventure. My childhood was marked by travel. At that time, at the end of the seventies, China was something extraordinary, an unknown empire with no entry permit for the Western world. My father was responsible for making sure that when a button was pressed, the processes were set in motion and, well ... steel is rolled. I know how to screw in a light bulb and I'm damn proud of it.

When we started the trip to Asia, I was about five years old and my sister was two. My father stood out unpleasantly at the baggage check at the airport. He had wisely packed a salami almost a meter long in one of the suitcases. We were aware that China would be a culinary, shall we say, adventure.

So-called jumbo planes were new, really big planes. My father was totally thrilled. Luisa and I were given wax crayons and coloring books, and the flight to Beijing took about 17 hours.

In the next few years we flew a lot and each time we combined it with really nice vacations. At that time it was possible that the company paid for Lufthansa flights and we quite cheekily booked the cheaper Singapore Airline. This way we had a nice extra vacation money. However, we also almost crashed twice. As a little boy, I didn't realize it, but as the tears ran down my mother's face, my coloring book became less and less important to me.

We made stops in Nepal and India. There I got to know the sacred cow. On arrival in New Delhi, a hotel with a sealed toilet lid in the room awaited us, but the poop had not been removed beforehand. Still, the employee demanded a tip. It was stuffy and hot. Near a river was an outdoor pool where all the local kids were happily splashing around. It was filled with brown river water and of course I wanted to get in on the action. I was very timid and the other children laughed at me.

Where there is poverty, there is faith. An urban prayer mill temple was imposing and I rolled some gold sculptures at the foot of the temple with my hand, this was part of a prayer ritual. My father gave a begging child a pen, the child's eyes lit up with joy. Next to him sat a begging man with black, rotten legs. So much suffering.

We flew on to Malaysia and the Philippines. Untouched nature by the sea, dreamlike. Even the accommodations looked like big coconuts. After only five meters in the sea I was surrounded by colorful shining corals. The locals performed almost naked dances on the beach for the few guests from the West.

Whenever we were in China, we spent a few days in Hong Kong. It was the Mecca of all children's dreams. So many toys everywhere, madness.

There was also a dolphin show in Kowloon, attached to a huge amusement and animal park. Luisa and I especially loved the big trampolines, where we bounced around for hours.

I liked the typical hotel smells, a mix of chlorine for the swimming pools and cleaning agents. Funnily enough, I also like the smell of gasoline.

The hotel in Wuhan (Central China) was built especially for us steel-rolling families from the West. We were shielded from the outside world. When we left the hotel complex, there was immediately a crowd of gawking Chinese around us. My blond sister with blue eyes even had her hair grabbed occasionally. Wuhan then was far from what it is today. Planned as an industrial city, it was still far from it in 1978. It was poor and dirty. The hotel area was now our new home. The men were driven to the steel mill six days a week in the morning and returned in the evening. The rule on the bus was that the old-established employees were allowed to sit in the front and the freshmen had to sit in the back. Women and children always waited outside the hotel for their return. In the old-fashioned way, the women took care of the children, and I don't think my mother was really thrilled about it. She did all kinds of things to keep everything in order, but actually she just wanted to get back to Berlin. She started crying when Luisa and I listened to a 'Heidi' radio play in which Heidi was homesick. That's when all the dams broke for my mom. She tried really hard, she even tried to bake bread. She didn't succeed very well, but she tried. I remember that even the stove once went up in flames.

Like in an agent movie, the incoming mail to us was read beforehand. So it happened that my father received congratulations on his promotion from the Chinese before he knew about it himself. We were under observation around the clock, we German 'Longnoses'.

There was a small, self-operated company pub. Posters of soccer teams hung on the walls and songs like 'No woman no cry' were played. It reverberated strongly out to the courtyard and my sister and I got to hear it all when we went to bed at night. The resident companies in the hotel included a Japanese company. The difference was very noticeable in the morning: The Germans were popping aspirin and the Japanese were at synchronized early morning sports on a field.

A popular destination was the Yangtze River, the longest river in China. It was about an hour walk there. We had to follow a small sewer. The earth was parched everywhere and had cracks because of the drought. There were water buffalo as farm animals and they made turds the size of tellermines. Occasionally, someone in our group was not paying attention and stepped into such a huge pile. The shit poured through the toes. For us kids it was interesting that there were frogs, fish and tadpoles in the waters. We passed small village communities on the way. They had cesspools, which were stinking manure holes in the ground about 20 square meters in size. You could have easily dumped a body there. Funny, why am I actually saying this now?

The Yangtze River is known for its extremely strong current. Once a year there was a swimming competition. From one side of the river to the other, the swimmers arrived at the other bank about 70 kilometers further downstream.

The bank of the Yangtze River was rocky, we watched passing ships and threw stones into the river. There were pieces of rock that held something like rock crystal inside. I collected those; it became a hobby of mine, I collected rocks.

There were spittoons in every room, on every corner of the building, all over the country. For some reason, the Chinese were constantly spitting. By now I guess it has been banned.

Often we were invited to official dinners, where there were such wacky things as sea cucumbers or even monkey brains to eat. Brains, for example, were eaten with a kind of straw cut in half lengthwise. You poked into it and then slurped the slimy brain mass. Rice with alleged chicken meat became my favorite dish, as I had no other choice. We tried to compensate for the vitamin deficiency with tablets.

The hotel was like a big adventure playground for us kids. We climbed up the hole-designed exterior walls and jumped from roof to roof. There was always construction going on somewhere and we helped ourselves to the building materials. Once I dropped a brick on a friend's head and it needed stitches. I felt very guilty.

The family took many short trips, including one to Shanghai. During the many sightseeing visits, I got stuck with some homemade ice cream from a street vendor and came down with dysentery, a dangerous stomach and intestinal infection that occurs mostly in tropical countries. I spent a full six weeks in the hospital.

There was a medical department in the basement of the company hotel. Surely the best that China had to offer at that time. All the children were afraid of it. It stank of iodine and the thick hypodermic needles were pushed into the bodies with a running start.

For the possibility of doing sports, there was a bowling alley, a ping-pong table and a gymnastic apparatus in the hotel. Once a soccer match was organized in the city stadium. Our men against a Chinese selection. The small, rural stadium was packed and the hotel won three to one. I was mighty proud of my father, he scored a goal.

The uniform in China at that time was blue or green, without exception. Students were recognized by a red neckerchief and their green caps had a red star on the front.

The company school was on the ninth floor and my way to school in first grade was the elevator. We lived on the second floor. All classes were taught in one room by one teacher at a time. My buddy with the hole in his head and I were the first class. I don't even remember the teacher's name, but it rhymed with vomit and so we called her in secret, Mrs. Vomit.

There was a party location, the so-called 'Old Hotel'. There, the men celebrated their frustrations off their chest. What was so special about it? The liberating mood. After all, they worked six days a week in a steel mill in China and were locked up in a hotel with their own wives. Of course, there was a lot of frustration building up. I always thought the parties were great.

When we left China again, I was sad. On the bus to the train station, people were already drinking in the morning and my father sang, »... aaaaahhh ... but the car, it rolls.« I cried, had completely forgotten Germany. Back in Berlin, I didn't know anyone anymore.

On our travels, my parents were always on the lookout for nudist beaches and every summer in my childhood we went to Corsica to a campsite called *La Vilatta* for about three to four weeks. The closer we got to our destination, the more hits from Italy and ABBA were played on the car radio. This was a tradition. My sister and I would fight in the back seat. Fortunately, Walkmans were invented and we put on those orange headphones most of the time and listened to radio plays.

At the campsite, people went to the supermarket naked, played tennis naked, and even sat at the table in the restaurant naked. I saw things there that I would rather forget. I didn't like it. The only evening event where clothes were worn was the disco every Thursday.

The nice thing was to make friends with tent neighbors, it was very easy. So every evening there was a nice round together. The campsite *La Vilatta* was a huge terrain with pools full of frogs and fish, a small pony farm and even a mini circus that performed twice a week. For my sister and me it was a paradise, except for the outhouses where we even had to stand to poop. We often went on excursions to explore the island. There was a river, I think it was called Cavo. It was very long, its rocks were just below the surface and quite smoothly washed by the current. We could sit on the rocks as if in a bathtub. All around was coniferous forest, an oasis.

I definitely had a very beautiful and exciting childhood. You can't get off to a better start than that. Strange what happened later in my life.

Teenager

China II

I was 14 when the family moved to China for the second time. This time I was taken right out of school and my circle of friends. The city of Benxi is just above North Korea and on the way there we took a vacation in Thailand. First we spent a few days in Bangkok, a full city with many sights, which we eagerly visited. We visited temples where monks lived. On river tours we saw how people lived on the shore in wooden houses built on stilts and how trade was done on hundreds of small boats in the middle of the water. It was impressive and all the pictures were memorized. Various animal enclosures were also there: elephants, monkeys and snakes. Every idiot goes to Thailand nowadays, but back then it was not like that.

The crowded streets of Bangkok were really busy, one small store next to the other. Very exotic food offers at every corner. Every third store sold pirated products, especially clothes and music cassettes. I bought a 'Best of David Bowie' cassette.

It was dirty and you could just about cut through the sultry air with a pair of scissors. My mother will certainly remember the bus tour to a snake show in the jungle. On one stopover, she sought out a small makeshift toilet and when she reached for the paper, a large, gray-haired spider jumped out. She screamed and ran out of the quiet restroom with her pants down. On the bus, there was unusual, colorful fruit to eat as a snack.

By train we continued to Hua Hin, a beautiful peninsula. A modern hotel resort directly on the sea awaited us. The beach was full of small crabs that first crawled into their sand holes just before my foot touched the bottom. I never caught one, they were very nimble. A little further from the hotel there were small local beach kitchens. For the equivalent of a German mark, we got a huge portion of whatever was there. We preferred not to ask which animal it was. A Fanta cost 15 Pennys and it was available in at least six different colors and flavors, completely sugared.

In the evening we ate at the hotel and there was always something special, for example ice sculptures at the buffet. Luisa and I even went to the disco once, where only little western music was played, some songs from Dire Straits were there. We had fun anyway.

I contracted a severe ear infection. The air conditioning in the rooms was set too cold. Off to a completely overcrowded hospital. There it stank extremely after medical liquids. On display on the shelves were pickled organs - even human embryos, eerie.

Our last stop in Thailand was Pattaya, then a place of sin. We were clueless. A busy road ran right along the beach and every other vehicle was a cab honking for passengers. There were really only three kinds of businesses on the beachfront: Whorehouses, bootleg vendors, and Thai boxing stalls. The hookers at the entrances kept talking to me, »Hey sweet boy, come in, have a look.« Desperate, I took my mother in my arms and pretended I was taken. Only once did I walk into such an establishment. There, Thai girls sat behind a big plastic screen with a number in their hand and the customer could choose one, two or even three girls for small money. In the hotel pool was often present an ugly German who always had three changing and scantily clad Thai girls around. From this I concluded that it was also possible to book by the day. I picked up somewhere that a hooker cost ten German marks per day and night. The male tourists sprayed their disgusting charm like in a very bad 70s porn.

At that time I was still very interested in martial arts and occasionally watched Thai boxing. I was sitting at the bar in one of those places, watching a fight, and suddenly a young Thai man was stabbed in the back right next to me. At that time Pattaya was a dangerous place. I watched a documentary on television some time ago. In recent years, many things have changed there.

Through private contacts, we came across a former GDR officer who had fled the country and offered unusual tours. He took us to the border region with Cambodia. My father and I went swimming under a waterfall in the middle of the jungle. I had to think of the movie *Stand by me* and was a little afraid of leeches. In a jeep we drove on to a gold mining village where we were offered emeralds and rubies at buying prices. We took a ruby necklace with us. A heavy jungle rain then chased us away. The second tour with the ex-officer took us on a small cutter to a deserted island. We swam ashore and the water was full of cat shark larvae, which were embryos floating around in the water in transparent bean-like containers. I had to be careful while diving not to accidentally swallow any of these capsules.

Then we continued towards China, onward flight to Beijing and from there by train to our destination Benxi. In the dining car, we realized again where we were. The old familiar picture presented itself to us: The Chinese slurped at their rice bowls with something meaty and simply spat the gristle and other tooth-resistant stuff into the center aisle. For the most part, we stayed in our compartment and played cards. The bedding smelled musty and dusty. I internalized the feeling of being a stranger very much. I've always had the gift or curse of perceiving everything to the highest degree, and my emotional memory is frighteningly good.

 On the other hand, the landscape we saw at the window was breathtaking: mountains graded into terraces of cultivation and rice paddies wherever we looked. Watching the rural people at work brought our mood back to where we had been ten years earlier. It wasn't as extreme anymore, but we were still stared at as if we were aliens and China had changed very little.

We finally arrived at our hotel. Certainly there had been no cleaning there in the last weeks and months. The mattresses in our rooms were damp and a biodiversity of insects and those who would become lived there. I have never had to enter such a filthy bathroom again in my life. Brown, muddy water ran from the faucets. My mother got a rash and I got lots of pimples on my face as a teenager.

The view from the windows of our accommodation unit extended to what appeared to be a ruin under construction and to the hotel courtyard. In this courtyard, mostly feathered cattle had their necks cut around noon. That ran still headless something around and later there was rice to it. Delicious. Due to the many years I spent in China as a boy and teenager, I had lifelong problems with my vitamin balance. Fortunately, there are women who find light circles under the eyes sexy.

There was a small pool table in the lobby of the hotel. The cues were simply sawed-off sticks, but still. We had brought a VCR ourselves, including the incredible number of five videotapes, including Loriot's skits. Loriot was one of the best german comedians ever. We watched the same movies every night, over and over again; we had nothing else.

One beautiful summer day, the staff plus family went on a trip to the mountains surrounding the city. It was finally a nice change of pace. When we got high up, we couldn't see Benxi. A brown smog cloud prevented it. China is dirty.

Again, we were invited a few times to official banquets, so we could again enjoy the culinary variation of Chinese cuisine of that time. No problem for the men, as long as Tsing Tao beer was also offered.

I was supposed to be sent papers from my school so I wouldn't lose touch. That didn't work, I lost the connection. However, we were only there for about three to four months. So it worked.

Once I was walking down the main street and at the end I came across a huge square, I mean really huge, Hitler-huge. I had my Walkman on and was listening to the live version of 'Don't you' by Simple Minds. Everything tingled in me, this size and in addition the live version, I got goose bumps.

In a department store at this place I learned that there was a discotheque in the building. Hard to believe: there was a fucking disco in this unworldly place. Two weeks later we went there in the evening, officially. We were seated like VIPs in an extra room behind windows.

They played Modern Talking exclusively, all evening long, over and over, no joke. What was interesting was that the joy prevailed. The Chinese just wanted to dance and have fun, it seemed to be new to them. On the circular, sprawling dance floor, women danced with women arm in arm, just for the fun of it. It was beautiful to watch. At one point I asked my sister to dance with me to 'You're my heart, you're my soul'. Somewhere above North Korea, quite an absurd snapshot. I'd be interested to hear what Tom Waits would have to lyric to that.

Occasional excursions were offered during our stay, for example, we visited the largest dripstone cave in China. There, my father had to use the bathroom. But the toilet cubicles had no walls and the bowls were separated only by a knee-high wall. Ever taken a dump when ten Chinese are grinning at you?

Otherwise, not much happened and eventually we headed back home. I will never forget how delicious a piece of decent white bread with butter and salt can be. That's what we got at the Holiday Inn Hotel in Beijing as an appetizer - can do anything.

Benni

Benni and I grew up in the same part of town, we knew each other through school and played in the same field hockey club. He was the coolest guy at school back then, I admired that a lot, I looked up to him. I was rather naive and still looking for my style. Benni had a lot of freckles on his angular face, reddish hair, he somehow had something Irish about him. Why Benni liked me as a buddy is a mystery to me to this day. He lived with his even cooler older brother Holgi in the house of his parents very close to the field hockey field of the sports club. Our parents liked each other and they occasionally met in the garden for a bottle of wine or something. Klaus and Ellen rolled their own cigarettes, seemed alternative.

We were around 14 years old when we had a free-for-all. We were sitting downstairs in the party cellar of the house and Benni found a bottle of Campari somewhere and mixed it with orange juice. I drank only one glass of it, Benni the whole bottle. Later, when we were back upstairs in his room, he wasn't really feeling well. He was crawling on all fours and when his dog suddenly confronted him, Benni said, »Hello Fuzz,« and threw up right in his very hairy but sweet face. Poor guy. Holgi then came home and helped cover up our mess.

Benni is a musician, he plays keyboards, back then he had a Yamaha DX7 synthesizer. His first band was called Major 7, I once heard them play in the parish hall of the local church, some of the choruses I still have in my ear. Today he plays in the Berlin band Goldfish.

I don't know why I have met so many musicians in my life, the only thing I know how to do is whistle and dance, but that's it.

By a strange coincidence, we both knew the actress Marion Kracht. On his bulletin board hung a heartfelt autograph from her, I think it said: For Benni, who has just as many freckles as I do. It was a small world back then in Berlin-Zehlendorf.

Then, in the summer, Benni, his parents and I went on vacation to France together. We planned a week-long canoe trip through the rapids of the Dordogne and a camping stay in Arcachon, at the sea in the southwest of France.

One two-person canoe each for the parents and for both of us. The water was cold as fuck and there were small caves in the high rock walls of the river. When you went in there, the water was icy. On our tour we often passed castles high up on the green hills beside the river. When a day was coming to an end, we would look for a place to sleep, preferably near a village so that there was a possibility of possibly finding a small supermarket. Sometimes we were lucky, but often we had to somehow make ourselves comfortable on the barren little stone banks.

Benni often sang while paddling, often it was Bob Marley's 'Redemtion Song'.

We didn't know that the Dordogne was like a V in cross section. On my birthday, we sat in our canoes and I ceremoniously got a wreath of flowers placed on my adventurer cowboy hat. We were close to shore and it was assumed that we could easily get out of the boat. To the shore side this was true, but I got off on the left side. It made blubb and on the water surface floated only my hat with the flower wreath.

Once we spent the night on a very small campsite, where there were also sanitary facilities. We had arrived quite early that day at our destination for the day and Benni and I explored the surroundings. To our delight we discovered a very small fair. At least there was something going on, for example you could ride a bumper car or shoot at targets with an air rifle. We did the latter and won a bottle of sparkling wine, which we drank with pleasure in the colorfully illuminated bustle of the fair. This special atmosphere has left its mark on me. I don't even remember if it was at the fair or at the campground, but there was a pinball machine somewhere, Benni liked to play those things. I stood next to it and he smoked a cigarette of the brand Peter Stuyvesant while gambling. I asked him if I could smoke one too. Benni was a little older than me and said no.

We now drove on to our next vacation destination, the campsite near Arcachon. Chris de Burgh was playing quite frequently on the car radio on cassette. I didn't find it that special there, but we settled in and talked a lot while playing cards.

However, I really enjoyed the occasional trips we took. I can't remember the name of the town, maybe it was in Arcachon, I don't know. After Benni miscalculated the placement of his plate in a pizzeria, he started trying to cut his pizza and the whole thing folded around the edge of the table onto his pants. We strolled through the small alleys, everything was set up like markets.

And then there was a concert there in the evening on a spacious field, quite barren, dark sandy soil. It reminded me a bit of the Middle Ages, maybe that was the motto. I don't remember, but I remember that Benni and I were on a slightly rocky hill and there were a few young people to the music always shouting »Deeestroy« to the music, heavy metal fans, I suppose.

Another night we went to find a disco. We only knew approximately where it should be. The path led through some fields with tall grass and the moonlight was very bright with a clear night sky. From a distance we saw some lights, which we then walked towards. It was again a fair, but it was larger and it was deserted, some lamps burned nevertheless somewhat helplessly and abandoned before itself. A few corners further we found the disco. To our surprise it was well attended and we stayed there for a while. On the way back, the night was much darker and we had problems to orientate ourselves.

Benni I have met over the years now and then by chance, mostly at parties, concerts or at *ClubA18*. In the social media, we still have contact.

The clique

Back in Germany, I was surprised when I saw my old schoolmates again. Everyone was suddenly smoking cigarettes and drinking alcohol at parties. Before, only Jan, Henning, a handful of other people and I had done that. What the heck, now it went right off.

All in all, I went to eleven schools.

- short break for applause -

I left one of the grammar schools with five Ds and an F in math and transferred to a less demanding school that was more suited to me. As far as math is concerned, I know the rule of three, the commercial interest formula and I can also add one and one together. That's all I've ever needed in my later working life.

I quickly established myself in the clique there and also had an instant crush. Her name was Karen and she was a straight-A student. She always chewed gum, smelled of it, and wore too big down jackets in the winter. The affection was mutual, but we were both much too shy and more than a one-time smooch after a party in front of her parents' house never happened. Both parents were teachers, I felt pretty stupid. I unconsciously took advantage of the fact that she was the best at school. She tutored me in French and also let me copy some exams from her. Nevertheless, I had to repeat the ninth grade. I wasn't stupid, I just had other interests. It was no different with

Karen. She would talk to me during tutoring and I would just stare at her, not really noticing what she was talking about. I think she noticed that too. I also think she kind of liked that.

For all the newbies: In the past, there used to be a half hour of blues in discos and at parties, around midnight. Perfect to ask a girl to dance. In my teenage years, songs like Richard Sanderson's 'Dreams are my Reality' or Berlin's 'Take my breath away' were played. Whenever Karen was present, I would ask her for a dance. Closely embraced, I smelled her gum and her hair as always. Oh yes, those moments in love. I will also never forget the blues dance with the girl with the killer boobs. I had to put myself, horny as I was, while dancing a little sideways, against it one is simply powerless at this age. More about her later.

The first couples formed, they felt grown up and acted a bit aloof. The boys and I were not ready yet. Sometimes I fear that I still am not and probably never will be, too much chaos in the head, no woman can stand that in the long run. But we were great at partying. We were the measure of things in the western hemisphere as we knew it. We stole records and cassettes at WOM (World of Music), but I was scared and held back.

Smoking cigarettes was not as outlawed then as it is nowadays. People smoked everywhere: In the schoolyard, in offices, even in sports clubs it was totally normal. It was forbidden on the subway, but nobody cared if people smoked anyway. On the way to parties, we were often subway surfers. The doors of the outdated wooden cars could easily be opened during the ride. We held on to the outside handles and enjoyed the thrill.

Most of my buddies didn't care about the lessons at all. Jan, Henning, Marian, Joe and I were always the center of attention and, as I learned, I can proudly claim that I was the top topic in the girls' room. Women always liked the boyish thing about me, I was never a tough guy.

Marian brought marijuana at a basement party of Henry. Of course I tried it, but nothing happened. I was told that the stuff would only work after four or five times. And it did eventually, but I didn't like the effect. I just got stupid in the head and giggled like an idiot.

And we messed up, my God did we mess up a lot. We often skipped school, instead we went on trips to Main Street, visited porn cinemas, hung out at the memorial chuch in Berlin or the Europe Center. When we didn't feel like going to individual lessons, we went to the forest next to the school and smoked marijuana. I, however, rather rarely, as you can imagine from my description above.

I remember that a new young and quite small teacher came into our class. She introduced herself in a barely audible voice, and Jan, Marian and I unceremoniously hoisted her onto a cabinet and left the classroom without saying anything. Of course, we were in trouble.

The Beastie Boys came out with 'You gotta fight for your right to party'. Jan, Henning and I didn't need to be told twice and we visited *The Power of the Night* in the City more often; a huge circus tent to party in. We sold small pieces of a leather belt as dope to be able to afford the entrance fee.

Jan lived right across the street from me. As I recently was told, he still lives there today. His mother unfortunately passed away and he inherited the condo. So it came to pass that one fine summer day we met early at 6:00 a.m. at the railroad tracks and plated a 12-pack of beer. We got through the first hour of biology class without any damage, but then we had bad luck. In English class Jan had to read out a text and he slurred his words. He was immediately sent to the principal. I didn't get caught, but Jan, the lousy traitor, couldn't keep his mouth shut. As punishment, we were ordered to participate in the school choir, which took place twice a week outside of normal classes. Fortunately, the prettiest girls in school were also in the choir. My voice was terrible at that time and I was assigned to the triangle. At least I couldn't do any major damage there. Lord knows I tried, but the triangle just wouldn't break when I smashed it against an amplifier in full rock 'n' roll ecstasy.

The choir tour

I was happily surprised when it was announced that a choir trip was planned and even Jan and I were allowed to go. The theater group was also going. Theater rather appealed to me and I voluntarily participated in it as well.

In two coaches we drove to Burbach, a small town somewhere in the south of Germany. Once there, we were horrified to find that the windows in the rooms and toilets had locks on them. Didn't work at all, and our first order of business was lock picking. I tried it with delicate dexterity, when that didn't work, Jan kicked the window frames vigorously without further ado. Not elegant, but effective.

The rooms were strictly separated into girls and boys. We didn't give a damn, at night it was like a train station. One woman (killer boobs) fell asleep in bed with me. We were awakened the next morning quite rudely by the otherwise liberal teacher. There were no consequences.

During the day we rehearsed and our favorite song was by Simon and Garfunkel 'Sound of Silence', this song still reminds me of the choir trip. Meanwhile, there is also an awesome version by the band Disturbed. In the theater group we rehearsed a 15-minute skit. I played a king with a cooking pot as a crown on his head. In the choir, I was promoted from triangle player to drummer. One night we were even allowed to have a party. Otherwise, we snuck out of broken windows, got drinks, and made ourselves comfortable outside in nature, even if it was cold. Oliver even came up once with a joint where the filter was a tampon, dangling from the blue string.

We visited a local church, how boring. But we spied a full case of Flensburger Pilsener right next to the altar. Strange, but it was. We waited until everyone had left the church, then grabbed the case and stole it. I think I'm still resented by him or her up there to this day. At that time, we were stealing for all we were worth. At least one of us always had a long coat on, the others distracted the employees and he packed up. Also popular was the 'two-for-one cigarette trick': you took two packs from the shelf at the cash register, reached into your inside jacket pocket to get out your wallet, leaving one box in your jacket, always worked.

One evening I was sitting alone with my buddy Alex in the room, everyone else was out. A small table, two stools, a candle and two six-packs of beer. He also had something going on with the bride with the killer boobs, a topic of conversation was found. We had a good chat. He was more of the sensible sort and a little older than me, but still available for all outrages. We understood each other very well. After a few hours we decided to hitchhike to London together this summer.

In retrospect, I notice that Alex had quite a bulbous nose. It looked like a pair of glasses sitting on top of a misshapen potato.

London

No sooner said than done. We met one morning with packed back-packs at the border crossing Berlin-Dreilinden. We had to go in the direction of Holland or France and after only half an hour we were given a lift. Back then, people were simply less afraid of picking up hitchhikers. We were euphoric and made good progress.

As we sat on our backpacks somewhere on the side of the road, Alex looked at me and said:

»Orange juice!!!«
»What Orange juice?«
»Orange juice!!!«
»Yeah, what...?«
»In the backpack!!!«
»So?«
»Broken!!!«

The tetrapack of orange juice had burst in his luggage and everything was dripping with sticky sugar stuff. No matter, we still had my clothes.

Around 7:00 p.m. we arrived at the Dutch border. It was raining, we were stranded at a gas station and had already resigned ourselves to seeking shelter somewhere and spending the night outside. We were sitting in front of the gas station restaurant with a sign 'London' in our hands. A guy came by and said we had to get to so-and-so - I forgot the name of the town - to catch a ferry to England. It wouldn't be his route, but he would drive us there. We got on and calculated that the trip meant a 150 kilometer detour for him, a bit scary. Alex sat in the front and had his Swiss Army knife handy in his pocket for safety. How ridiculous, he probably would have just hurt himself with it or it would have slipped out of his hand and hit me right in the forehead in the back seat. We were skeptical and slightly nervous. However, it turned out that he was just a very nice Dutchman. At night at 11:00 we caught the ferry quite barely and exhausted. We bought two cartons of cigarettes in the store, Alex Camel, I Rothmanns.

We found out that you can't smoke and yawn at the same time.

Still in the dark we arrived in Dover. Within 24 hours from Berlin to England, record-breaking. In Dover, however, we were stuck for six hours, no one took us with them. At 12:00 noon, we finally reached our destination. We took the tube to get to central London, up the escalator and we were in the middle of a noisy, protesting crowd. We just walked along, everyone was very friendly. For fun, for example, we shouted, »Yeah, right.« After half an hour, we noticed that it was a gay and lesbian demo and we sat down in a café.

We were very tired and asked people for a campsite. Abbey Wood was recommended to us. Okay, another hour and a half by slow train out of London City, but we arrived. It was a large, lush green and empty campground, we set up our sleeping spot, drank some wine and listened to the 'Rocky Horror Picture Show' and Sting's album 'Nothing like the sun'. It started to rain and we finally went to sleep. Alex read me a chapter or two from the cult book *The Hitchhiker's Guide to the Galaxy*.

We visited many famous places in London during the day. I found it a bit dull, only the legendary Virgin Record Store, that excited me, music excites me.

At the campground we noticed two girls about a hundred meters away from us as the crow flies, we wanted set them straight, you know what I mean. One evening the two were not there and we, buzzed in front of our tent, had the stupid idea to do something romantic. We placed a lit candle on an empty candy box in front of their tent. I guess they came back late at night and what was left was a blob of wax on a cardboard box. The next day we waved to them with a bottle of wine in our hands and there they came by. As I said, we were a hundred meters away and from a distance they looked good. It turned out that they were very boisterous, fucked up and certainly not good looking english girls who eventually drank away our wine and liked to give Alex hefty pats on his arm. The next day we decided to leave - so everything quickly packed up and off to Dover.

We were almost broke, we could still afford the crossing to Calais. Once there, we checked in again at a campground. In front of us at the reception was an older couple. The receptionist made a mistake, thinking we belonged. She pressed a tent number into our hands and waved us through. While setting up the tent, my postal savings book appeared among my stuff, I had forgotten it. 500 Marks - saved. To the bank, to the supermarket. It started to rain again. Alex had bought, among other things, a bottle of Malibu, disgusting coconut-egg liqueur-something. Comfortably we squatted in our tent, the rain splashed on it and Alex slurred constantly: »Maaali-BUH« and got wasted. Sting and the Rocky Horror Show were playing in the background again.

Later we decided to go to the local disco. It was only moderately crowded. They were playing 'Stay on these Roads' by A-ha, among others. I will never forget the mood I was in, as corny as the song may be. Alex had ordered a whiskey-cola and not half an hour later he felt sick and threw up all over the toilet. We rather went back to the campground, sleeping. The sound of pulling a tent zipper always brings back fond memories of my childhood.

A carnival was set up on the main square of the small town. No visitors, as if emptied, spooky. We sat down in a fast food joint and rewrote a choir ride song 'Sentimental Journey'. The lyrics written on a napkin went something like this:

»Gonna make a journey to Great Britain
How does it feel to hitchhike in the rain
Got no food nor money to buy it
But it took our hearts away
Money, our biggest problem was the money
And honey, all we ate was just honey«

After a week the 500 marks were almost gone, we had to go home. We didn't want to pay for the camping site, so we climbed over the wall at three in the morning. It was cold as hell. At the place with the fair there was also a church, rather a ruin. The church bell was on the ground and offered an optimal hiding place for our backpacks. We had to hold out until nine in the morning, when the first bus left. We squeezed into a phone booth to protect ourselves from the cold and lit a warming candle. Somewhat misplaced, we took a nap.

We bought tickets for the bus that would take us towards the highway. We still had some money left. Cigarettes or something to eat? The choice was not difficult. We thought the way back to Berlin would be as fast as the way there. But it took three days and we had nothing to eat. Every time we were dropped off at a gas station with a restaurant, we waited until people left their table and pounced on the leftovers.

In the last section of our return trip we were lucky, a totally stoned Beetle driver took us to Berlin. Pink Floyd never sounded so good.

Nicola

In Berlin, Alex had three girlfriends going at the same time. He was a bit overwhelmed and I had to lie on the phone to manage everything. I felt like a boxing trainer in the ring corner, fanning his protégé with a towel. He was leaving for America for a year. Among many others, all three girls were there for his farewell, and he waved from the car with a fat grin. When I noticed that the questioning eyes were now looking at me, I made a hasty exit, mentally dodging bottles, eggs and apples.

Shortly after, Alex, 19 years young, died in a diving accident in Florida. He was a guy you were sure could do anything. I liked him a lot and firmly assumed that he would become a successful architect or something like that. I still think about him a lot. I hope he's up there waiting for me with a glass of »Maaali-BUH«.

Before he passed away, we went to a garden party. It was a beautiful summer and my parents were away for three weeks. On a wooden staircase facing the garden, I met Nicola. Either she was bored, drunk or she found me attractive, we got talking anyway. Her stepbrother was a friend of Alex.

After an hour we kissed. I had nothing like that in mind, she just grabbed me. I had nothing to object to as a silly, horny teenager. Let's call a spade a spade, I was horny as the neighbor's dog and she was a vamp. I think that sums it up.

My first steady girlfriend, my first great love.

Mrs. Gräber was the blueprint of a vicious teacher. I had French and German classes with her. She wore the same clothes every day, everything in beige and light brown. The entire class had to stand up to greet her and call out in unison, »Good morning, Mrs. Gräber« loud and clear. She always had a ballpoint pen in her hand and kept drilling it into her wrinkled cheeks. Her flabby arm fat flapped back and forth as she wagged her finger around, and I was exposed to the sight of her armpit hair.

Once a week she would summon me to her office, even though I hadn't done anything wrong. She just enjoyed putting me down - which she succeeded in doing. At that time I was still very shy and insecure.

Teachers either loved me or hated me. As it turned out, my biology teacher hated me, even though biology was my favorite science subject.

My friends and I wandered around the Kurfürstendamm and in the Europe Center a couple of guys hit on our companions. The girls found it fun and played along. Jörg, Marian and I were pissed off. It ended up that we were beaten up, we were outnumbered.

Apparently said biology teacher was nearby and claimed to the police that I had been the culprit. A few days later the phone rang, I answered it and was told that there was a charge of assault against me.

The stupid bitch reported me. I swear I didn't do anything.

However, I could participate in a theater project organized by a social worker, then everything would be okay.

A theater provides the perfect stage for mentally disturbed people. Largely egomaniacal and narcissistic actors experience a family of plays (wait, what does that say about me?). There's drinking, there's drugging, and everyone craves admiration and validation. Everyone wants to upstage the other.

The first play I was in was called *Hooded*, and it was about left-wing demos, which were still the order of the day in Berlin-Kreuzberg in the '80s. There was the so-called 'Red and Black Front'. The band Ton, Steine, Scherben was an integral part of the left-wing scene in Berlin. On stage I played a left-wing autonomist, which no one bought at my young age, it was just ridiculous. We also performed the play once in a correctional facility, and the inmates laughed themselves silly at us.

The second play was already better, *Noah's Ark* at least made it into the newspaper and we had a nice troupe together. It was about a test run in a nuclear bunker, where different characters clashed.

Meanwhile Nicola was my girlfriend and when we were in the theater workshop together, she was asked if she would like to play alongside me. That's how Nicola and I ended up being hired for the two-person play *Burning Love*. This time it was not directed by the head of the theater, but by an external couple. The rehearsals were a lot of fun and we received something like a little acting training. Memorization was never difficult for me. When I graduated from senior high, I simply memorized two Leitz folders and ended up with a grade point average of A-. All the medication makes it harder for me nowadays. The play *Burning Love* was about a love affair in which both of them passed each other by. In the end, it was doomed to fail. We even had a two-hour interview with the BILD newspaper and a big photo of us was published, right next to smaller articles about Michael Jackson and Gerard Depardieu. My 15 minutes of fame, I was recognized in the subway.

At least we got consistently good reviews in some newspapers, we even made it to Sat.1 (TV station) breakfast television. Our performances came to an abrupt end when the head of the theater stole away with the box office, a pity really. Story of my life, always on the verge, never the big breakthrough, I like to think of the scene in the movie *The Fisher King*, where Jeff Bridges is drunkenly talking to a Pinoccio character and basically says the same thing. In hindsight, it turned out that the boss of the Kreuzberg theater had a thing for little boys.

In the basement of the theater lived a mother cat with three young kittens. When everything went down the drain, I took a tomcat with me, he lived to be 21 years old and became my faithful companion over all those years.

I had a 180-square-meter old apartment all to myself. No idea what my parents had in mind, but they left me alone during their vacation. In the large living room, Nicola and I put two couch pieces together and gathered all the quilts we could find. I had episodes of *Alf*, the movies *Apocalypse Now* and *Planes, Trains & Automobiles* on video, but that was incidental, we were otherwise occupied, you know. She had also pierced my ear and hung a silver bat on it. I had neglected the apartment a bit, so to my amazement a sunflower grew out of the kitchen sink. I think it was from spilled hamster food. I'm not particularly gifted when it comes to household cleanliness.

My parents returned from their vacation, opened the apartment door, looked a bit disturbed and closed the door again. They took refuge in the sports club and gave themselves the edge. Nicola and I indecently followed them and entered the bar room in the club. Me in a black coat, black dreadlock cap, with a silver bat on my ear and black kohl pencil around my eyes. She in a black miniskirt, black suspenders and a tousled blonde mane. Unforgettable how all the jaws of those present dropped at the same time. It was similar at the Schlachtensee, a lake, in the circle of friends. No other woman presented herself on the lawn in suspenders, even then I had the talent to choose striking women. Or they picked me out, hard to say.

Nicola's father did not like me at all. When I introduced myself to him by name, he only replied, »Never mind, it can happen to anyone.« He continued to stare at the television, where a film with Klaus Kinski was playing. »The boy can not even decant a bucket of water« and other niceties I had to listen to. At that time he was probably right, I was just a good-looking but very naive boy, nothing more.

Within a very short time Nicola had changed me completely. I think my father was a little proud of me. That my mother was happy about it, I dare to doubt.

Nicola had a bittersweet sense of humor:

You know those little plastic egg cutters with the wires? Yeah right, she woke me up one morning with that: »Get up!« *ching, ching* and grinned menacingly at me.

Or in the bathroom - we often showered together - she would casually say, without looking, »Will you hold the towel for a minute?« And she hung it on my expectant manhood.

One evening we were sitting on a bench by a small pond. I babbled some sappy romantic stuff for ten minutes to impress her and after a while she said:

»Man, do I have to take a shit.«

We had a kitschy Garfield annual calendar in which she always wrote all kinds of things. Once a week it said, »Love you, honey.« But also other things, such as: »For the second time from behind«. This little bitch.

And she had shoes, lots of shoes, and perfume, lots of perfume.

Just recently I got her number from her stepbrother. I think she lives in Hamburg and until now I didn't dare to call her. The last time I met her was in 1998 in a schoolyard. By chance, we had finished our High school diploma later at the same time at the same college. I thought I wasn't seeing straight ... what the fuck. After eight years, she's just standing there looking as stunning as ever. We didn't talk much, she wanted my collected newspaper clippings from our theater days for an application and of course I gave them to her. Advanced Economics and Performing Arts were my favorite classes. At the premiere of a play, she was among the audience. I knew that and was grotty with nervousness on stage. Actually, I wanted to impress her. I had the role of Don Juan and had written my own text.

A woman who played a nun asked me one evening after a performance in a disco if I would like to have a threesome. I declined with thanks. With two women, okay, but with another guy, nope, no fucking way.

Nicola's foster family was intellectual, educated, alternative and very nature-conscious. Her stepfather gradually accepted me and told me about Brecht, Weil, Klaus Hoffmann, Edith Piaf, Jaques Brel, and so on. He taught me a few things casually, of course I was much too young to internalize it all completely, but some course was set with me. Often there were small concerts in the garden behind the house, I enjoyed them very much, but did not tell anyone. Culturally, Nicola's family was just very different and I let it all sink in attentively and quietly. Thank you for that.

Nicola had a small room with a rickety bunk bed. When I met her, she was very vulnerable, yet she was confident and strived for security. She found my family and became a little absorbed in it and I was a part of it.

After her I was no longer shy, she knew things about my body, holy shit. However, she determined our relationship, so I had to brush my teeth after every cigarette and I was not allowed more than two beers at parties. Also, I was allowed to cut her fingernails and pluck the runs out of her pantyhose, I was quite under her pistol, I must admit, but I learned a lot during that time with her, as a teenager. About women, for example.

Nicola grew up as a foster child. As far as I know, her mother was a prostitute and her father had shot himself in a phone booth while on an LSD trip.

She has two brothers, Phil and Flo. I became friends with Phil. He even got together with my sister for a short time. He was a goth, he had dyed black, highly toupeed hair, he was thin and pale, and he was into The Cure and Sisters of Mercy. The other brother, Florian, was three years older, very sensible and family-oriented, and as far as I can remember, he had only one girlfriend, Michi, in the two or three years we knew each other. After almost 25 years, I was able to contact him again on Facebook. He has a family with three children and is a France fan, all as planned. Good thing.

France

Phil was with Yvonne and I was with Nicola. In the summer we wanted to go to the French Côte d'Azur together. We men were adventurous and hitchhiked, our girls would follow two weeks later by train.

This time I was the older one in the hitchhiking team and was more experienced, but that didn't matter. Somehow we would get down there, we thought.

And it started off really well, on the first day we made it to Orange, France. Around 8:00 p.m. we arrived at a gas station and decided that it was enough for this day. We bought two bottles of red wine and sat in the scenery in front of the entrance. Three hours later we had a buzz and looked for a place to sleep in the dark behind the gas station. The next morning we found out with booming skulls that we had gone to sleep on a generously laid out garbage dump behind the gas station. Phil had puked on his thermal mat during the night. We now smelled of that certain something and made only very sluggish progress in France. The next day we lost patience and took the train for the rest of the way to Antibes. I liked the small train stations of southern France. There were two campgrounds in Antibes and both were hopelessly crowded. We were not allowed in.

Phil and I dragged our luggage to a beach bar and ordered a few bottles of beer. As life sometimes goes, a 30-something-year-old Frenchman walked by and approached Phil. Where do we come from, where do we want to go and what kind of music are we into? We talked a bit and without further ado he invited us to his house. His name was Franck, yes with ck. He worked as a bus driver and just like Phil he was a Goth. He had a nice little house with a large stone terrace and reeds as a half-height interior wall covering in the rooms, very cozy. His girlfriend Marie also lived there. She always opened her bottle of beer with her teeth and laughed hysterically in between stories. I liked her. I just like weird personalities. We were allowed to stay, there was enough room.

For two weeks we went to clubs and parties together and barbecued almost every evening on the dark red paneled terrace. What a summer! Of course, it didn't work out at all that I didn't really look like a goth, and Marie fixed me up: highly toupeed hair. It didn't look so bad, I now felt like I belonged.

After two weeks we picked up our girls from the train station, they were also allowed to move into the summer house. But it was no longer the same. Of course we also had fun, game night fun. There was a cool theme party a few houses away, everyone dressed like in ancient Rome. In sheets and sandals we danced until the sun came up. In between, first Yvonne and Phil, then Nicola and I withdrew to a side room for sex.

One of Franck's buddies drove an orange Citroen 2CV. He had a police siren in the car and occasionally he used it, for fun of course. On the last day of our vacation we went to a fair. It was hard for all of us to say goodbye. Of course we exchanged all the info about each other, but we never saw each other again. We were aware that it had been a special time. Our relationships didn't really harmonize on this vacation, as is sometimes the case in couple vacations. I realized that traveling alone was my thing and I did that for many years.

When Phil and I on the way back, again as hitchhikers, from France crossed the German-Dutch border near Aachen, two policemen approached us, identity check. They asked us where the journey should go ... »Berlin«. They took us to the police station, where they searched our backpacks. In my rolled up thermal mat they found a hash pipe. It was Phil's, the bastard had hidden it with me. What the fuck, I was pissed off. I had to go down to the basement with one of the cops for a physical search, that means including: »ass cheeks apart«. It was extremely uncomfortable and I think the fucking cop even had fun with it. Thanks a lot for this experience, Phil. They didn't find any drugs, we were allowed to continue our trip.

Through vitamin B in the sports club, I was able to arrange for Nicola to train as a nurse, including a room in a nurses' home. She had a very small bed in her room, I slept on piled coats and jackets next to it on the floor. At this point, she had taken all the advantages for herself from our relationship. I was beginning to realize that she didn't need me anymore.

The doorbell rang at my parents' house and Nicola was facing me. She looked at me very differently than usual, somehow defensively, at a distance, as if she had something to confess.

»I want to break up.«

Ouch. Petrified, I stood there and closed the door without saying anything. Strangely enough, I was relieved, but also completely perplexed. At that exact moment, the starting gun went off. My heart broke, but now I could do all the things that had been denied me before - rock 'n' roll. The excessive life began. I loved her very much, but on the other hand I had been looking at other women for a while, I'm just a man.

She had probably met a 20-something who was a bit more mature than me. His name was Micha and of course I hated him. She was always one to look for what would get her ahead in life. I no longer met that standard. Women drop you when they get bored with their toys.

For about three months Sophie was my girlfriend, a sexy piece of DNA. I had always had the hots for her, she was a fan of the Doors and the Rolling Stones and always compared me to Jim Morrison. I guess that guy was her ideal of a man. I wasn't at that musical level yet at all. She had beautiful, laughing eyes and, as they say, a mischievousness about her in her eye - plus boobs to adore.

Weeks before, we, that is, some friends, me and also Sophie, sat together at a campfire at the lake Krumme Lanke lake in Berlin. It was a warm summer night and we wore so-called prism glasses from the optician. If one had smoked some weed or had thrown an LSD trip, an awesome optics. At that time I was still with Nicola. I was fooling around with Sophie on this little sandy beach and it was actually already clear to me that the breakup with Nicola was imminent. So it was already foreseeable and it hadn't really surprised me, yet it was the closing point of my teenage era and it felt important and tragic.

Portugal

At the same time my sister ended her short relationship with a certain Lars. We got along well and it seemed, no, it screamed to do something together. Lars and I booked Interrail tickets: for 430 Marks we could travel by train across Europe for a month. Before that, we had a week's vacation at my parents' apartment. We took advantage of that, of course, and partied with some friends every day. We built empty beer bottles like dominoes strung together in the apartment, through every room of the 180 square meter apartment. With beautiful stucco on the ceilings, by the way. In Berlin Bel-Air.

Always at Christmas, we sat in the corner room facing the crossroads, ate fondue and then played cards. I remember that very fondly. That's family, that's nice.

I left a week earlier, heading for southern Germany, to earn some money from my parents' acquaintances in a sports mat company. At that time, Saddam Hussein had just invaded Kuwait. I was working in a factory with the son of the boss and was mourning my relationship with Nicola a bit, I was lonely and slept on a camping couch in the office of the factory. It always smelled like those rubber mats. I spent the evenings listening to love songs. It was just a week or maybe two days longer, it felt like a whole month.

Then it was off, Lars arrived and we decided on the Holland-France-Spain route, with Portugal as our destination. We had a lot of fun on the way there, even met friends from Berlin on the train and two compartments full of Italian girls who were really up for anything.

The slow trains in Spain were especially vagabond-like romantic. Our feet dangled from the train at the boarding steps and we enjoyed the scenery. Depeche Mode came out with 'Personal Jesus'. Music, wine and these vast, gorgeous landscapes, some cute Italian girls who had the hots for us, an absolute sense of freedom.

Arriving in Lisbon, Lars was stupid enough to ask someone for weed right at the train station. He followed a guy into an alley and was robbed. Money gone, ID gone. We had to go to the german embassy to clear everything up. The clothes we were wearing stank terribly, our feet were black with dirt and I was really annoyed.

First we had something to drink, so we went to a tavern. We ordered tequila and were surprised when we were served two long drink glasses. The barmaid poured and did not stop until the glasses were full to the brim. We were told to say stop when pouring, apparently that was the custom here. Completely drunk and somewhat haphazard, we stumbled back out into the midday sun.

Again, we happened to meet friends from Berlin, they had rented a cottage for the summer, in the middle of nowhere. In a shabby old VW bus without sliding door we drove there. After a day at the beach on the Atlantic Ocean, we had dinner together by a fire on the terrace. After several bottles of red wine, Lars got the idea to light his farts. Sounds shallow, but it was fun. A real competition started and the women present just rolled their eyes. I did not join the fart orchestra.

Lars and I slept on the floor in the large main room of the house and, as we fell asleep, heard a female voice from next door shouting,

»You loser!« Someone had probably drunk too much red wine and the cravings of his girlfriend were probably no longer particularly important to him in this state.

Back in Berlin, I celebrated my birthday on the large lawn at Berlin's Schlachtensee (lake). I had decorated the whole lawn with tea lights, it looked like a landing strip. I had invited 40 friends, 200 came. The Schlicht brothers were on an LSD trip and were pushing a primate movie. One of them bit my buddy Sonny and others in the nose. The idea of two freaks on LSD lurking in the bushes biting people's noses to satisfy their hunting instincts was completely absurd, but hilarious.

'Teenager in love' by Dion and The Belmonts didn't make it onto my playlist now, that time was over.

Bread & Games

I grew up in Berlin-Zehlendorf, perhaps the most beautiful district of Berlin, I just say. The Schlachtensee was right on the doorstep, lots of nature. That meant: rubber dinghy in summer and ice skates in winter.

There is a student village in Zehlendorf with about one thousand housing units. It has existed since the 1960s and is a listed building. There's the *Club A18*, a legendary student pub. I've been going there since I was 15 years old. It was only four years ago that I had to give up this connection; my manic-depressive excesses were my undoing. I had applied to be the new manager and put myself in excessively, too much, there was a backlash and I withdrew. I'm only a rare guest now, about once every three months for karaoke night.

Those were great times back then at *Club A18*. The parties in the circle of our clique started at 9:00 p.m. and often didn't end until 9:00 in the morning. I had a large circle of friends and there was always something going on. We met almost every day and everyone just worked along to keep everything going. I had a habit of putting together mixtapes. At least once a week I would bring one in and annoy the bartender on duty, but they liked the music. Often I was the DJ at parties.

After all-nighters, we occasionally had breakfast on the roofs of the student houses in the summer. Life was good.

I started writing poetry and song lyrics when I was 16, not well, but I enjoyed it. I've always been fascinated by what words can trigger in the reader, what moods are conveyed. For example:

Silverwine   **Sweat**   **Thunderstorm**   **Cello**

or very simple

Nicotine   **Ozon**   **Cancer**

The Band

The woman with the killer boobs knew about my passion for writing and also that I had gained some theater experience in the meantime. She in turn had a new boyfriend, Ben. Ben was three years older than me and a musician.

Ben wanted to put together a rock musical, and the woman with the killer boobs found in me a lyricist and choreographer. Until then, my musical range was limited to bands like The Cure, Sisters of Mercy, The Police and Depeche Mode, i.e. rather dark music.

We met regularly at Ben's house. At first there were only three of us, Ben, Frank and me. Ben and Frank already knew each other a little. We sat together, drank red wine, chatted about women and exchanged ideas about music. Occasionally the two grabbed their guitars and played. This was all new to me and I thought it was great. Frank was a huge fan of The Beatles, he had 15 different versions of 'Strawberry Fields' on record, and Ben was on a Doors and Stones kick. I entered the musical hall of fame. Ben became my mentor, so to speak, and I admired him. He told me stories about The Rolling Stones, such as how they had to fulfill a record contract and recorded a song called Cocksucker Blues as revenge. Keith Richards had all his blood replaced for 50,000 $just to relive that feeling from the first Heroinkick. That's the kind of stuff he told me. A few years later, I happened to meet Keith Richards in a bar in Venice, and yes, I wouldn't put it past him.

Frank had a sense of humor all his own, sometimes getting up in the middle of a conversation, going to the door or a window and talking to people who weren't even there. A bit weird, wasn't it? At that time he was someone who accepted only originals. Fashion or music, only original from the 60s or 70s, a new pair of jeans or corduroy pants couldn't be cool. I saw Frank and Ben again at a concert the other day, after 20 years. They played a song from our old rock musical and Ben even mentioned me in front of the audience. I was surprised, reacted spontaneously and went briefly on stage after the song and hugged first Ben and then Frank. Ben could handle it, but Frank looked at me completely irritated when I thanked him. I believe that with real buddies, time shouldn't matter. You stay that way all your life, even if everyone has gone their own way.

What should our rock musical be about? We agreed that it should be a failing love affair. Ben introduced us to 'Duke', a musical work by Genesis. The record still inspires me today, especially when writing.

After such an evening Frank and I stayed overnight, to the left and right of Ben's bed lay a mattress each. I started talking in my sleep, Ben woke up. When I was finished and shut up again, Frank agreed with me and mumbled »Yes, yes, yes, yes ...« into his pillow. Thereupon I gave again something to the best and Frank answered again: »Yes, yes, yes, yes ...«. This went on for about 15 minutes and Ben sat in the middle of the bed, completely baffled. The next morning he told us about the nightly conversation.

We christened the rock musical *Maurice*. Casper joined us, he was supposed to write lyrics as well. After a few months Ben and Frank had written some songs, but it wasn't about that anymore, it was about our friendship. The musical was never finished. We made big plans, our two musicians tinkered with their bands The Out and The Moods and I was always there with full zeal. Unfortunately, I couldn't play an instrument and my voice wasn't that special at that time either, with nervousness it somehow didn't work. Acceptable singing was only possible when I didn't care about other people's opinions.

Casper wasn't with our rock musical for long, he lived in his own strange world and his thoughts were hard to follow. When he became homeless, he moved in with my parents for three months and slept a lot. He was interested in figuring out his dreams. He had an old Renault and one night we drove down the highway to the city to celebrate. The next morning he had an epileptic seizure and we took him to a hospital. He hadn't taken his medication. If this had happened a few hours earlier, on the freeway, good night. He then soon moved out again and I never heard from him again.

I always thought the bands' gigs were great, I was a kind of roady and helped where I could. Frank and Ben founded together first The Circus and then later The Ground. A small fan base formed, which always came to the concerts. I designed flyers and small concert booklets with the song lyrics and some poems of mine. One of my poems was so somber and sad that Ben's mother cried when she read it.

War broke out in the former Yugoslavia and Ben and I sat up all night in my room at my parents' house in front of the TV listening to The Doors 'The End' non-stop. For us it was the first real war we witnessed and we stared at the TV in horror.

It was the beginning of the 90s, bands like Nirvana, Pearl Jam and Soundgarden founded grunge rock. Dirty, rocking, destructive - brilliant. We felt backed into a corner and we didn't care.

Many people associate the 90s with Dr. Alban or LaBouche, for example, terrible music. No, it was the rebirth of rock, excessive and brute. Especially the songs 'Smells like Teenspirit' by Nirvana and Pearl Jam's 'Alive' were absolute firecrackers. To this music we could spray all our excess energy on the dance floor. At *Huxleys*, the DJ even played just those two songs for an hour once, Ben and I danced through it. I've always been a passionate dancer, as a teenager I often danced for six hours straight.

The woman with the killer boobs organized a New Year's Eve party and some musicians from our clique performed there and covered 'Smells like Teenspirit'. The party was still too fancy-schmancy for us. At a little after midnight we decided to leave, grabbed a bottle of whiskey and took the subway to my house to continue partying.

Arriving at Schlachtensee station, I had the completely wacky and over-the-top idea to undress and dance naked on the street. That's what we did and passing cars gave horn concerts, it was cold as fuck. Those were the first moments that were striking and indicated mania. There were three of us: Ben, Sonny and me. Why the two of them went along with it, I don't know, but I've always had the talent to inspire other people for even the most absurd things. Around 1:00 a.m. we arrived at my parents' house. I assumed that they were still partying somewhere at this hour. I Thought. We turned the music up loud. Lenny Kravitz was playing and suddenly my mom was standing in the room and Ben and Sonny were somehow trying to hide their nakedness behind chairs, which they failed to do. All in all, a very embarrassing situation for the two of them. I thought it was amusing.

In retrospect I have to say it was a legendary New Year's Eve and I still have to smile when I think back on it. My mother certainly does too.

In the middle of the city there was an - what do you call it? - Event, happening, an exhibition. Anyway, it was about the music of The Doors. In an old, abandoned industrial complex on the river Spree, artists set about transforming rooms into songs by The Doors or even poems by Jim Morrison. For ten marks admission, we walked through these rooms as through a self-contained universe. Dramatic, the last room: drop axes swung from the ceiling to Morrison's spoken text 'Rock is dead'. After an hour, sliding metal doors opened as large as if a ship were being launched. To 'L.A. Woman,' the view opened onto brightly lit Berlin, a subway train passing by. I had a tingling in the stomach area and goose bumps. Now I understood the music and Morrison's words, I was gone for the time being.

I had read in a book that Jim Morrison did not wear underpants out of conviction. I had to try that out, with the result that during the test week I always had to travel at least three subway stations further because I couldn't stand up. Well, free-swinging in a train that jolts back and forth, that's sometimes enough at that age.

We had a lot of contact with other bands in the Berlin scene, worth mentioning would be Peter Fox from the band Seeed, with whom we played together on some concerts. Even then it was clear to me that he was very close to a musical genius, he had real power.

There was a girl band, The Lemonbabies. They had the bad habit of swapping instruments on stage during a gig. In the midst of all the band hullabaloo, I met Anne from that group. After a gig, she came along to Ben's apartment. Mr. Jack Daniel's was making the rounds and Anne ended up on a mattress with me. We made out, but she didn't want to take it to the extreme. Irritated, I went to sleep. Hours later she woke me up and whispered in my ear that she wanted to have sex with me after all. I slept on. The next morning I saw Anne's feet peeking out of the bedspread, which was at least a size 12. I was then the subject of an issue of the band magazine Lemonpress, but I never met her again. I still sold her my Gibson Les Paul guitar, which I had never played.

Road trip to Munich, Fürstenfeldbruck. A friendly band had invited us to play a gig at a concert. Without further ado we packed instruments, amps and a pallet of beer into the band bus and hit the road. It took us two hours to get on the right track, Ben was a lousy driver. A guy named Chris and I sat in the back of the van and gave us the edge. When it started raining, I had to fill in as windshield wiper, it was broken. I shimmied out the passenger window and used a cloth to clear the view.

We arrived in Munich much too late, it was about 11:00 p.m.. When we entered the concert hall, we were welcomed and announced directly from the stage. There was no time to set up the equipment, we just had a jam session together. Drinking, pissing on the walls of houses, getting caught and disturbing the peace of the Munich suburb.

I woke up in a white fur coat on a couch and didn't know where I was at first. After breakfast, we hiked up a mountain. Why we did that, I do not know. After a really rockin weekend, we drove back to Berlin with me again as the windshield wiper.

The apartment-share

When I had once again gone too wild in Berlin, my mom kicked me out of the apartment. I called Ben and asked him if he could use a roommate. He said yes and within three hours I was moving in and out. After only a few days, my parents felt sorry for me and my dad brought us a food package.

Ben and I renovated my room while listening to good music and every night when *Al Bundy* was on the new channel *RTL*, we paused and laughed our heads off. Even today, after 28 years, I still enjoy watching the Bundys, a classic.

I bought my first CD player, invested a large part of my earnings in new, interesting bands such as Soundgarden, The Black Crows or Element of Crime.

Ben said to me that it was my turn to wipe the surfaces of the kitchen cabinets, after all, he always does this. Besides a sticky layer of dust and grease, I found a porn magazine from 1974 and had to clear away quite a few wine bottles in the shape of the World Cup. You always got a free bottle of wine after the tenth order at *CallaPizza*, left over from the 1990 World Cup. So much for him always cleaning up there, lying bastard. But that's just how he is, when nothing else works, just lie brazenly.

He was once in the hospital, a gastroscopy was pending. The two nurses were very attractive and he denied the question about anesthesia. He wanted to come across as cool and ended up gagging and throwing up when the tube was inserted. He stood there as a complete idiot, but at least he had left a presumably lasting impression on the pretty ladies.

The *TIP city magazine* was an integral part of our apartment-sharing magazines, as were *Rolling Stone magazine* and *Musikexpress*. So we always knew what was going on in Berlin and in the music scene. The current issue of the Social Democrats newspaper *Vorwärts* and one of Charles Bukowski's works were always on the toilet.

I was sitting on my mattress in my undershirt one evening, eating ravioli from a can, drinking a Radeberger Pilsener and watching TV. Ben came into my room with the current issue of *TIP* in his hand and pointed to the cover without saying anything. Pictured was a man in an undershirt eating ravioli from a can and drinking Radeberger Pilsener. The title read: »Poverty in Germany.« Wordlessly, Ben closed the door to the room again and I stopped chewing for a moment and looked irritatedly into the can of ravioli.

Ben and I would often listen to audio dramas quietly in the background to fall asleep, something like *The Three Question Marks* or Ghostbusters *John Sinclair*.

Often the bailiff was at the door for Ben to seize things. Ben would just bring anything of value, guitars and amplifiers, into my room, the cuckoo was not allowed in.

One night Ben and the woman with the killer boobs came home, I also just came from a party, was hungry and found a single fish stick in the freezer. I sat down on a chair right in front of the stove and put the thing in a pan. It burned despite my stare and hypnotic gaze, I was just too hoe. The woman with the killer boobs watched the situation and couldn't stop laughing for two hours. Oh well, besides, I was naked.

Ben had caught a nymphomaniac in between, for a whole week they did not leave the room. According to Ben, she said to him that she wanted to try something new. She said, »Insult me!« Ben's comment to that was, »You doofus.«

For a while, out of conviction, we didn't have a TV in the shared apartment, Ben and I decided to dabble in philosophy instead. We read Nietzsche, Sartre, Rimbaud and Co. for about half a year. We noticed that, contrary to our expectations, it didn't do us much good and we ended up buying a new TV. From a purely philosophical point of view, Al Bundy's wisdom simply could not be surpassed.

Hot town, summer in the City

Ben and Frank had motor scooters, which I thought was super cool. I also made an attempt to buy one second hand, but it was stolen from me again the very next day. I think they were the same people I bought the scooter from. We didn't take it too seriously with the traffic rules, it happened that we rode three on one scooter and did without helmets. My enthusiasm for these vehicles has lasted until today, I still ride scooters. A car is too expensive for me and I no longer have a wife and child.

Since Ben was on a Doors trip, he wanted to get as close to Jim Morrison as possible, even on the outside. He went to the barber to have a light perm done. That day, he subsequently showed up at band rehearsal looking like Tony Marshall, with lots of little tufted curls. He also wore a light blue frilly shirt and looked bleakly at us with his bloated face. What a laugh we had.

A running gag was to often sing Happy Birthday in bars when Frank came in. The other guests applauded, stood up or even sang along. He didn't like that at all.

One Thursday, Ben and I planned to party at the *Far Out* disco in the evening. In the afternoon, we went shopping at a mall. When the post office ATM confiscated Ben's creditcard, he freaked out and unceremoniously kicked the whole thing together, quickly gone. It was summer, we were in a good mood, bought a few beers, sat down in front of a store, drank and had a great time. Time passed quickly and before we knew it, it was evening and we were off to the *Far Out*. Ben tried to casually prance down the stairs to the subway and really laid into it. As a pack of girls walked by, he immediately jumped back up, stroked his hair and tried to look good. He must have been in serious pain.

A concert was coming up and we started a promotional campaign. After work, Ben and I collected the guys with the band bus. We drove mainly in East Berlin from pub to pub and asked if we could put up a poster. The later it got, the longer we stayed in the bars. At each stop, we also drank a beer and chatted with the staff. As time went on, the posters hung more and more crooked and in places that made less and less sense. At around 3:00 in the morning we stayed seated. Two hours later we realized that we had lost Ben. We searched and found him in the men's room. He was sitting on the toilet with his pants down and his head was leaning against the wall. He had fallen asleep while taking a shit. Since we were no longer roadworthy, we called the woman with the killer boobs and she picked us up. Enthusiasm looks different.

Mike and Olli

Mike was one of the dopeyest guitarists I've ever met. He liked to smoke pot a lot, and you could tell. I remember an evening with the gang in the living room of our shared apartment. There were five of us, sitting around the coffee table, drinking red wine and intensely philosophizing about God and the world and these ... what you call th ... yes, women ... thanks.

Mike was wearing a frilly orange shirt, 60s style, and sitting huddled on the sofa. He was completely stoned as usual and didn't say anything for probably two hours because his head was in neutral. The rest of us argued fiercely. In the middle of the conversation, he suddenly rose from his lethargy, indicated greatness with a raised attention please finger, and took a deep breath. Everyone was quiet now, staring intently at Mike. He exhaled with a long sigh and slumped back on the sofa. Somewhat stunned, we took note, Ben grasping his lowered brow in mourning.

He had also met our drummer Mirko once to give him the band room key. Mirko came all the way from the south of Berlin, Mike from the far north. They met in the middle, an hour's drive for each of them.

»Well?«
»Yes what?«
»The key.«
»Ahhhh, shit.«

Mike was also one of those who nodded into a phone receiver and then said he'd said yes.

Olli was in the band on the organ. I remember we were downstairs in the band room and heard a thump. Olli was punch drunk, had abruptly stopped singing 'Honky Tonk Women' and fell down the stairs. His purple sunglasses were hanging crooked on his nose and he was screaming »Rock 'n' Roll!«.

One morning he woke up and could no longer feel his legs. As it turned out, LSD deposits in the spinal cord were causative for his condition.

The whole band and I visited him in the hospital. Six rockers with bottled beer in their hands, horrified looks from the nurses. Olli was happy about our visit, put on his bathrobe and on the way out he played 'Once upon a time in the west' theme on his harmonica. We just walked past the intensive care unit. He also had a black walking stick with a silver skull as a helper. That had some style to it.

Once outside at the main entrance, Mike first rolled a joint. Olli warned us that he would probably pass out if he smoked something, but that the nurses would know. And so it came to pass, after only one deep drag he simply slumped over.

A few days later I smuggled him out of the hospital in the evening and we went to rock out at the *Fun House*. In the morning at 3:00 a.m. I brought him back, the security guy of the hospital was well-disposed towards us and didn't betray anything. Olli had gotten him some weed beforehand.

The biggest gig of the band was in the refectory of the Technical University of Berlin, an audience of about one thousand people was waiting for us. We were nervous, especially Frank. He had probably drunk a whole bottle of whiskey before the gig and was then in good spirits. However, he didn't really have his bass under control anymore, but he thought he would play like a young god. Ben was really pissed off. After the last song Frank slurred something about encore in the backstage area. I've never seen Ben angrier, he was very close to punching him in the face.

The company

My parents suggested that I could go ahead with my vocational bac-
calaureate. That's how I ended up enrolling at a special school for
economy they have here in Germany. I didn't care, but I had to do
something. The school was far away, a long bus ride every day, and in
the meantime I was exclusively occupied with music.

In order to obtain the collage degree, it was planned to complete
a one-year internship alongside school. That didn't make any sense
to me, an internship wouldn't do any good. I would just be a cheap
laborer, assigned to the most menial tasks, a yawn from a resume
point of view. Nevertheless, I had an interview at Dr. Gerlach Ltd.,
a real estate company. I explained my view of things to the boss and
asked without further ado for an apprenticeship opportunity, not an
internship. The boss was a friend of my father's from the sports club,
and I had also known him from an early age. I decided to train as a
commercial clerk in the real estate and housing industry. Actually,
I was only interested in satisfying my parents, none of this really
interested me.

Then, in September 1991, it all started. I started in the accounting
department. At that time, I didn't even know how to fill out a bank
transfer form. What I did know was that in the Monty Python movie
Jabberwocky, the word 'accountant' was used as a swear word, rightly
so, as it turned out. Twice a week I went to vocational school and I
had to keep a training record book. Everything I had worked on was
to be documented in it. Since I always had to do the same shit, my
creativity was in demand.

I was warmly welcomed into the company, everyone was very nice
and for me it was the first time I had worked in an office. I had just
turned 19 and was still pale green behind the ears. It was a very
young team. I felt a kind of sense of optimism. The company was
doing well and so were the employees. I was assigned an instructor:

Mr. Staller, a tall, thin chain smoker with a scruffy-looking five-day beard, authorized signatory of the company. I noticed that he always beat around the bush with me. He always seemed a bit nervous and distracted and never got to the point. I had the feeling he wasn't really on the ball. His behavior was strange.

After only two months, Dr. Gerlach sent me by plane to Frankfurt. I took part in a seminar in a hotel. It was about real estate financing through life insurance. I was completely out of place. What was the point? I wasn't the least bit interested. I was surrounded by business people and watched them. A strange breed of people.

I often got coughing attacks during sales presentations by our bosses. It was so dry and I felt uncomfortable in a room with so many investment advisors and associates. I would often leave the room, cough, and have to overcome myself to re-enter the room.

When I looked at our notary during a contract certification, how he supported his wrinkled ear area with his fingers, I felt quite different.

The company was right on Kurfürstendamm. Convenient, after work I could go out or go shopping and a friend of mine lived only five minutes away. Her name was Tina and she was a Messi, her apartment was overflowing with all kinds of stuff. There was hardly any getting through, but at the end there was a huge red bed in the shape of a heart. The first time I spent the night at her place, there were popcorn scraps all over it. She was a pothead and occasionally I would take a puff of her joint. I visited her frequently on my lunch break and we had fun. One winter day her mother passed away from an asthma attack, I left the company Christmas party to be with her.

The number of employees in the company was manageable, about twelve people. Lunch was usually ordered and we ate together in Dr. Gerlach's office. This did not happen without reason; it was always a working lunch as well.

Immediately after German reunification and the fall of the Wall, the boss brought Mr. Sommer on board. He was knee-deep in the real estate business of the former GDR, he knew all the important people. A smart move on the part of the boss. However, Mr. Sommer had such a bad saxony accent that I often had to stifle my laughter. I couldn't resist parodying him occasionally. I was a bit of a clown in the company.

Dr. Gerlach was a clever strategist, but he lacked the ability to interact socially and emotionally. He was aware of this, however, and made up for this deficit with material gifts. He didn't think much of me, but he realized over time that in my own way I also had some influence in the company, albeit minimal.

The company grew very quickly, champagne was often served at lunchtime and the annual bonuses were immensely high, even I little runt got a few extra marks. Once a year, the staff went on a company vacation together; we traveled to Budapest, Vienna, Venice or Istanbul, for example. It was always great fun.

We had seminars, lots of seminars, about communication techniques or memory training. Nothing technical, it was more like stupid drivel from a mental trainer who was charging way too much money for that shit. Within the company, it was always emphasized that every employee should be able to cover all specialist areas. Everyone should be able to do everything and be universally applicable. In the real estate industry, there are a lot of specialist areas; it's practically impossible to know everything.

Professionally, I wasn't a great light, but informally, I had something going for me.

What was new was that I had an income and the first thing I did was buy a pair of snakeskin boots for 500 Marks.

Mr. Staller had the idea to give me a dictation machine, what a bull-shit. I little freak should dictate something to a secretary? It disappeared in a drawer.

Greece

From May to July, I hung out at Schlachtensee lake. Girls were busy painting their bell-bottom jeans and exchanging bracelets. We guys provided drinks and music. And there was the stoner section. As indifferent as they felt, they were indifferent.

The Doors, The Beatles, Led Zeppelin, Janis Joplin, Jimi Hendrix … a magical summer.

The question arose, where to go on vacation. My buddy Jeppy and I settled on Naxos, Greece as our destination. For fun, we created flyers. Everything meets for a big party at Agia Anna Beach on Naxos. We distributed them at Schlachtensee and Krumme Lanke lake and within no time all schools and universities were informed.

At the end of July, we were off to Greece. Our group was to meet at the airport exit in Athens. I was traveling with Lot Polski Airlines, in a very robust propeller plane. I had an eight-hour layover in Warsaw, and in the hangar I met two friends from Berlin. We just plated two pallets of beer, AC/DC was playing loudly and the travelers in the airport were anything but taken with it.

I woke up in the airplane with newspaper around me. The stewardess looked at me not exactly friendly, I had probably let me go through my head again and now wanted to know if the food was already served. Her facial expression told me I should rather keep my mouth shut.

Arriving in Athens, I found my people at the exit of the airport, wrapped in sleeping bags. A few bottles of wine and cookies were lying around.

Boarded a shabby bus, to the port. Lots of backpackers, waiting for the next ferry. That dirty, oily harbor smell passes for romance with me. Up the steep stairs in the ferry, conquer a sleeping camp on deck, pick up overpriced sandwiches at Dimitrios and drink wine. A Julia then shagged in an on-board cinema, it was empty. There was a time when I had 15 Julias in my phone book, no way to tell them all apart. I had to lurk for clues on the phone in conversation.

Agia Anna Beach was an insider tip, miles long with wide dunes. There was a small campground with showers, the Maragas Camping-ground, but we took over or built our own reed tepees in the dunes on the beach. Occasionally military helicopters flew by menacingly close over our heads. They were trying to drive us out of our tepees and into the hotels. Every evening there was a big bonfire in front of a remote dropout taverna. I asked for LSD for my buddy Howie and me. We were given UFOS, papers. Papers are like little stamps, you put them on or under your tongue. I went swimming in the night black sea. The next morning I woke up, somewhere in the sand, Howie was lying next to me asleep and a big black bug was crawling out of his mouth. I felt very free. How to describe an LSD trip? It's magical, a vision and a monster. You feel energy, people, lights, and if you're lucky there are some nice visual effects to go with it.

There came the party weekend staged by us. Jeppy and I were sitting on a wall, it was about 5:00 p.m. . Buses came from the port, many buses, very many buses. All of Berlin came. We didn't have to do any-thing else, just watched. Hordes spread out over the beach. Guitars and bonfires everywhere, we were proud.

The author Richard David Precht must have been there, too, I just assume. I read his book *Who am I and if so how many?* It begins with

Naxos, reed huts and how he found philosophy. It must have been that night.

On another vacation to Greece, Howie was with us again. We were sitting on the beach on Paros in the evening and he had magic mushrooms with him. Well of course I took some and a really wicked trip ensued. We walked from the campsite through nature. Bushes became dinosaurs and stone walls became ancient Greeks hugging each other. We approached a small town among the hills and even from a distance I could feel the lights and the people. I walked through energies. We sat down in an open-air restaurant and ordered cocktails. When the waiter came to collect, I didn't know what he wanted. A friend then helped me with it. I had forgotten what money was. Then we went to an open-air disco, with a tree sticking up from the middle of the dance floor. To me, it looked like an alien monster rising from the bowels of the earth. What a visual.

I still spend the summertime on the Maragas Camping on Naxos every year.

Candy

I couldn't skip vocational school very often, I usually got caught and then had to come up with excuses. I tried to avoid my instructor, Mr. Staller, as much as possible. Every conversation was unpleasant for me. He wasn't the teacher type, could only impart knowledge with difficulty and in a roundabout way.

During the breaks, I kept seeing a very pretty girl in the corridors and courtyard of the vocational school. At that time I was into dark red hair, no idea why, but quite a number of acquaintances had this hair color. The vocational school also trained travel agents, unfortunately I didn't have any classes with her. During a boring school day, she approached me in the hallway. She was a singer in a band and invited me to a concert of hers. She had also just sung a radio jingle. It was the rewritten song by the 4 non Blondes 'What's going on', which she proudly played to me in her car. Her ex was the guitarist of Big Light, a Berlin band that had two mediocre hits.

After the concert and an after-show party we ended up in our shared apartment, Ben had also hooked up with a pretty girl and we sat together in the kitchen for some time. Ben and I gave it our all to impress them. He tried his extensive knowledge of music, I went for philosophy. I think the two girls were a little smarter, or at least more experienced, than we were. They thought our efforts were just cute, both stayed the night - won. I assured Candy that I was up to no evil and she had to grin because it was just off the wall. I seemed too harmless.

Candy lived high in the north of Berlin, in Spandau, together with a roommate. If I wanted to visit her, it was always an hour and a half's drive there. I remember that Ben and I were broke as usual. In the fridge there was basically a bottle of Jack Daniel's and a carton of cigarettes, but mostly nothing to eat. We were hungry. I called Candy and asked if we could come over, it was early evening. We set off on our way. Candy and her roommate Steffi cooked a ham and noodle broccoli casserole. Ben and I practically inhaled it, we were that hungry.

I was once invited to Candy's parents for coffee and cake. Their house was almost an estate, I did not quite fit into the picture. As usual, I was in my leather gear, smoking cigarettes without a filter, and look-ing a bit out of place in other ways as well. To make it perfect, the lid of the coffee pot came off when I wanted to top up Candy's mother. Right on the blouse, bummer. Still, there was a happy ending for me: down in the laundry room, Candy and I had a blast, but I chafed my knees during the action. It got a bit weird when she gave me a blowjob and wanted to kiss me right after, which I refused. She was astonished about that.

She used to call me Pinocchio, I suppose because I wasn't always about attendance at school and truth in general.

She had a hat fetish, dozens of hats hung on the wall in her room. Through Candy I learned about the bands Beggar's Opera, the West Coast Pop Art Experimental Band, and the hit songs of Manfred Krug. Her perfume was patchouli.

We were walking along a canal in Berlin-Spandau on a beautiful spring day. We talked and also got closer on a human level. I enjoyed it. Once we went to the *Fun House* in the evening and as usual I danced for hours and rocked the night away until dawn. She didn't like it, she was looking for something else. She realized that I was far from adulthood. She was right about that.

We were on the subway and she was planning her birthday party. I asked her what I could do to help. She said, »I don't want you to come.« A little puzzled, I looked at her and very slowly realized that she was just breaking up with me. I guess I was just a little too immature for her, I could understand that. Not so bad, I wasn't that much in love with her.

Through family connections within the band we had a gig in a small village, somewhere in northern Germany. Parts of the Dr. Gerlach GmbH accompanied us there, a long weekend to relax. We partied for three days straight. At the gig, I stole a four-meter-high inflatable dinosaur from the neighborhood and carried it on my shoulders through the village. I reached the stage and staggered around, everyone laughing. The next morning I woke up next to an accountant. I knew nothing more, fortunately neither did she.

As part of my training, I had to do an internship at a property management company for three months. The company was located at the Anhalter Bahnhof train station, which was more than an hour away for me. I had to check in at the time clock at 7:00 a.m. It was winter and I had trouble getting up. To work in the dark and back home in the dark. I came up with something. I took a time plug and plugged in a power strip, to that I plugged in a vacuum cleaner and the coffee maker. At 5:00 a.m. I was awakened by the noise of the vacuum cleaner and the coffee ran through. I usually listened to The Beatles or Cat Stevens for early morning chills. It was also somewhat contemplative in a strange way, I liked the quiet when everything was still asleep.

At a little before six, my train started. Most of the people on the train were returning home from a party, cleaning ladies coming home from work, and homeless people looking for a warm place to stay.

I ended up in the accounting department of this company right at the beginning. I sat together in a room with a woman of about 70 who read *Frau im Spiegel* or *Gala* (women's magazines) during her lunch break. It was so dull that I liked to go to the bathroom for a long time to somehow get the day over with, counting the minutes.

The vocational school class went on an educational trip to Wüns-dorf. We were supposed to look at the former Russian army quarters, no idea why. I only had this new band Nirvana from Seattle in my head. In the evenings, my fellow students and I hung out in the station pub, and after curfew we hung out in the lounge for a bit. I slept in public on the couch in the main hall for a week, everyone else in their rooms.

Little by little, I brought the band boys into Dr. Gerlach Ltd.. In the temp room, we had all the freedom in the world, at least in the beginning. Ben, for example, would take something somewhere with the company bus and come back after five hours with a new hairstyle and a shopping bag from the record store.

Due to the party, we suffered from a chronic lack of sleep. The work table in the room was huge, and often one of us would lie down under it with a screwdriver in his hand and take a nap. Now, if some-one important came in, we'd nudge them with our foot and they'd gasp, »Yeah, yeah, I'm getting it.« And waved the tool around.

Actually, it was never real work. We just met there, did something, listened to music and chatted. Through the job and the associated acquaintance with Mr. Staller, it came about that Mr. Staller financed a CD from the band.

We all noticed that he always acted a little strange. We assumed that he was gay, which in itself is perfectly okay, but in the trainer-trainee relationship I didn't feel comfortable with it, and not without reason. During a lunch break, he invited me to a restaurant for dinner and announced to me, visibly tense and at the same time in joyful anticipation, that he was gay. I answered to him that I knew that. Completely perplexed, he asked me how. I had to tell him that it was actually known to the whole company. It became clear to me why he never got to the point and always printed around so strangely - he was horny.

In the real estate industry, people are always celebrating, and Dr. Gerlach Ltd. was no exception. Mr. Staller drank a lot and sometimes it happened that he lost control and slurred things like:

»When I wake up in the morning and think of you, I get a boner.«

For a few months I had to move into his office due to lack of space. I suppose he had set that up. I sat across from him all day long, my office desk was made of glass. Whenever he was on the phone, he would look at me. It made me uncomfortable.

At a celebration at the sports club, he said to my mother, »I love your son.«

I was young, slim, handsome and had long dark hair. At that time, very often gay men were eyeing me.

I explicitly ask not to misunderstand me. I have absolutely nothing against gay men, but at the time and in my situation it was simply unpleasant and I could not handle it.

At a weekend seminar in Potsdam, there was another big party and Mr. Staller followed me to my hotel room. I tried to avoid him somehow. I started rearranging the furniture and destroyed an antique lamp, later I grabbed a plant in the hallway and hurled it all along the corridor. I rebelled against the intrusive stress. I ended up sitting on a closet and he finally left. Upon checking out, the otherwise friendly hotel clerk said, »This room would be something to talk about.« Fortunately, the boss paid for the damage done.

At the end of the year, at the Christmas party, the employees always worked on a gift for the four managing directors. In contrast to my day-to-day work, I put a lot of effort into this. I can be creative.

As a thank you for financing the band CD, so to speak, we produced a song about the company. Ben and Frank played the music in the studio, I wrote the lyrics and sang. We designed a nice cover and the bosses were happy about it.

Pretty much at the end of my time at Dr. Gerlach Ltd., I really hit my stride, I shot a twenty-minute film. Observation has always been my strength, so I made fun of everything I noticed in the company. I worked on it for over a month. A handful of colleagues and I recorded the lyrics after work and a business partner edited the video on the computer in his studio. It was a huge success and I was very proud of it. Mr. Staller said to me the night of the Christmas party after the screening, »A different kind of intelligence.« Well, thank you too, am I otherwise stupid or what?

In the end, it was all about finally putting this shit behind me. I passed the written exam without any problems, I had probably unconsciously memorized some things. However, the teacher for accounting and law, Mr. Borne, hated me and intentionally let me rattle through the oral exam with a single point. Forty-nine I had, fifty I needed, that stupid fucker. He was the kind of guy who couldn't make it in the private free ecnonomy and ended up as a teacher.

Wild at Heart

There was a time when I always woke up somewhere else, with some woman I had met the night before. I roamed around in clubs with filthy toilets and over-postered walls. It was my Sturm und Drang period. Once I woke up in a squatted house deep in East Berlin. While I was still dozing off, my new acquaintance said, »When boys are sleeping, they look like angels.« I escaped from that run-down house and it took several hours to get home, partly because I kept falling asleep and taking the subway back and forth.

I tend to look for girls who are a haven of calm for me. Full-bodied women have this calm aura for me. The feminine attributes are very pronounced. I'm emotionally unstable myself and usually can't be a rock in a relationship, although it does occasionally happen that I give off a balanced impression. I don't really understand that - must be the medication, the rest is acting. I like intelligent women.

My therapist thinks that I had little grounding in my childhood, which makes perfect sense. We were always on the move in the world, without any real grounding. Perhaps that explains my increased desire for security. My parents will certainly have a completely different opinion, they are also right. We were and are a great family team. It may be that it was only a short period at a vulnerable age that shaped me.

For most people, my preference for round women only evokes head-shaking, but over the years this has increasingly gone right up my ass. I credit my father for always being very tolerant: »Let the boy have his happiness.« And as is usually the case, you can never please your mother. None is good enough for her son. There was only one woman who ever accepted her, Sonja. Ironically, we were actually just friends, not lovers. That was probably the deciding factor, because she couldn't hurt me. She always called me 'cookie'.

My father once told me in a conversation at the counter in the sports club: »Your wife must always also be a friend, a life companion.« Today I know that he was right about that.

Basically, I find people who can enjoy or even indulge in an addiction much more interesting than the functional corpses that make our world oh so livable. Every abnormality has a story that needs to be explored. That is life, that is exciting and instructive. Mostly just such people are enormously gifted in many ways. I think whoever learns in life and can enjoy, has a good chance to be happy.

Gradually, manic behaviors began to appear in me. After a night of partying, I was completely overexcited on the way home. Henry drove us home in his white VW Golf. The car had a sunroof, I climbed out while driving and sang The Doors' 'Break on through'.

At that time, I would lie down on Kurfürstendamm at night because I was sure that nothing could happen to me. All the cars swerved and honked. A friend dragged me off the street and took me home, I was completely out of control. She cried when she realized how desperate I actually was.

Drug excess

It was towards the end of my training. There was a summer party at the sports club. A former classmate was also there. He had ecstasy pills with him and offered me one. I was curious and took one. After half an hour I felt fantastic, happy and was in love with almost every women who were there. Of all the drugs I know, MDMA suited me the best.

Even on the way to the *Rock it*, a legendary Berlin rocker Disco, you were approached by dealers on the street between the hookers. I now took advantage of these offers and got myself cocaine or speed on the way to the Club, why not? I didn't care, I wanted to have fun.

My vocational school buddy Mathew and I went to the Berlin *Love Parade* that summer and we were on fire, it was great. I danced in the streets - well, actually I rather jumped around in ecstasy.

Mathew knew someone who dealt in pills and powders. We could be there for purchase prices. Every weekend we went to the *Linientreu*. At that time, it was a techno club and drug temple. I took everything that the market gave, mostly ecstasy or speed, all mixed up. That was certainly very dangerous, but I was immortal.

Mathew always had to keep me from marrying some girl completely high. I was always head over heels in love on MDMA. One night he didn't succeed and I ended up on a farm in the middle of nowhere. I remember how the E in the car gradually wore off and the woman behind the wheel got uglier and uglier. I wish I had listened to my buddy. Thankfully, he picked me up the next day.

In the months that Sonja and I lived together, so to speak, we spent most of our evenings hanging out on my mattress watching movies. I think I had the last TV in existence without a remote control.

Our song was 'Creep' by Radiohead.

There was a Truck snack bar on the corner, where I often went to get a bottle of wine or a hamburger. Even though it was very cold, fashion-conscious as I am, I put on boxer shorts, sneakers and a coat, nothing more. Style – I´m good at.

Sonja and I were at a lame party in Berlin-Kreuzberg. Someone had E's with them, we each took one and met up with Ben's band at a pub, completely off the rails. I think that night I said something bad to Ben, it led to the break of our friendship. I don't remember what it was.

Sonja was so high that she peed her pants. I gave her my jacket so she could tie it around her waist to cover the mishap. She hadn't really noticed all that.

Our drug rush had to be financed, we bought from our acquaintance and sold on. I had a so-called 'ticker', that is someone who sold drugs for me. His name was Thorsten. He always ripped me off, I wasn't much good as a gangster, which in retrospect was a good thing. I should have smashed his face in, but I didn't. Consequently, I was taken advantage of. Every weekend, Mathew and I were on drugs, and that went on for three months. I had just failed my oral final exam, I didn't care about anything. I weighed only 134 lb at 6 ft, physically I was not well. The last I heard from Mathew was that he had been caught on a train at the German-Dutch border with 15,000 ecstasy pills. I don't think even his rich parental home could help him there.

A friend from the drug scene approached me at the *Linientreu*. She had an LSD paper with the nice title 'Comic' and wanted to exchange it for two ecstasy pills, no problem. A paper is about one third the size of an ordinary stamp and was drizzled with liquid LSD. Strictly according to the user rules I first took half, after an hour nothing happened and I threw in the other half as well. The girl in question came up to me again and asked me how much I had taken, a quarter was quite enough for someone who takes it often. The paper was double drizzled. So I had put 8 times the regular dosage under my tongue.

The look on her face said it all, I was screwed.

An unprecedented LSD trip followed, it started and got heavier and heavier. I understood God and the world and took off into galaxies that no human being had ever seen before. I got scared, higher and higher levels of consciousness, everything made sense. Would I ever come down from here again?

The *Linientreu* was set up like a circus arena. People on speed or ecstasy ran or danced around the dance floor in the stands. Due to the drugs they felt an enormous urge to move and as a consumer you dried out, the corners of your mouth turned white and you constantly licked your lips. My situation got worse and worse and I started having violent hallucinations on my rounds around the arena. Suddenly everything was full of bawling, raving Nazis, but only in one half of the rondel, the other side was safe, very strange. My fear of Nazis manifested itself in hallucinations. I hate violence, I hate stupid people who don't even make an attempt to mend their ways.

I sat down and the woman who had given me the paper reappeared with me. I asked why she was crying. She was not crying, I looked into her soul. I slumped forward and slapped my knees to keep from losing consciousness. I needed to get out into the fresh air and I didn't know how. I needed help, she refused and was still preoccupied with the fact that I had seen her crying. I found a dude to accompany me outside, it was early morning. My body was failing, more specifically my circulation. Death grinned at me with its ugly grimace, if you will. I tried to stay awake with cold water on my neck and biting into lemons and not just keel over. People's faces turned cartoonishly colorful and it felt like my brain was burning up. Hard to imagine, but it did. I was aware that I could die at any moment, but I fought and won. I was lucky.

Mathew brought in a pretty fucked up guy and we drove to his apartment. He showed us photos of a deceased neighbor, eaten by maggots, and he said that he never wanted to end up like that and decompose in his apartment because no one would miss him.

This was now the perfection of my horror trip.

But it gets worse than that. About a month later, my ticker Thorsten brought LSD mics, very small brown pellets, about the size of the pellets in a fountain pen like we had in elementary school. It was the weekend and with a razor blade I split the pill in half. I took one and threw myself into the nightlife. At 4:00 a.m., I still felt no effect, so I threw in the other half, too. That was a mistake. I went to the *Linientreu* faithful, it was 7:00 am, no effect at all. But then suddenly it kicked in, just not in the way I expected. No optics, no trip. Simply, my body was failing. I was a prat, deathly afraid again. Luckily I had been exercising from a young age - I think that saved my life.

I went home and was panicked. I put myself under an ice-cold shower to stay conscious. I opened the apartment door so that I could rush into the stairwell in case of an emergency. I didn't want to call an ambulance, then I would have had to admit to having taken drugs. After several hours of struggling, I couldn't do it anymore, so I rang the neighbors' doorbell. Someone on the third floor opened the door and I told him what was going on. He and his wife took care and gave me a vitamin cocktail and a coffee. He proudly presented me his record collection and actually put on 'Sweet child in time' by Deep Purple. That was absurd and I could not cope psychologically at all now.

After about three hours with the neighbors, I felt a little better. I went back to my apartment and lay down on my mattress, completely exhausted. *The Flintstones* were on TV.

The deceptive peace did not last long, suddenly the second half of the pill took effect. What the fuck.

I was already completely burned out and I realized that I now had to muster even more strength to survive. I called a friend, once again a Julia. She came over and I told her about my situation. Didn't she understand my condition, no matter, I needed someone just in case. We took the subway to her place. I had to concentrate or get excited about something very hard non-stop to stay conscious. The life and death struggle went on until the next morning. Then the drugs finally wore off and my completely exhausted body was functioning in stand-by mode again. It was the worst day of my life so far. Because of that I got a damage to my heart, since then I can't do heavy sports to my heart's content, I got heart rhythm disturbances.

A few weeks later, I finally let go of drugs. It was a very intense experience, but I regret it and can only advise everyone to keep their hands off hard drugs.

I made the mistake of lending my cell phone to a drug dealer. He was kind enough to accumulate 800 Marks in debt. To get out of my maxed-out overdraft, I took an additional job in the evening at a video store. Let me tell you, that's where you meet people. The big ones were the customers who disappeared straight into the XXX section, didn't show up again for a long time, and then still rented a porno plus an alibi movie, mostly science fiction or horror. The bad thing was that I always had to clean everything, and in the porn area it stank disgustingly. The store was on Kantstraße in Berlin-Charlottenburg, and some Hertha BSC soccer players were regular customers there. I thought that was great, of course.

The three months of excessive drug use took its revenge. I had the feeling that my soul was hanging crooked.

I developed severe depression. In retrospect, of course, I wonder to what extent the drugs had an influence on my mental problems. I don't think they had anything to do with the underlying illness, but they will have given me a little slap in the wrong direction. It took me a year and a half to get a feeling for rock 'n' roll again.

I am sometimes not sure if people pity me or are afraid of me.

Our acquaintance always wrote down by name who had bought how much and which drugs from him. I was also listed in his notebook.

The doorbell rang, not many people visited me. I was skeptical and first looked through the mail slot. I heard, »Oh, crap,« and a second later my apartment door was broken down. Five police officers with guns drawn and a German Shepherd stormed into my apartment looking for drugs. I was in shock. They found nothing, although there was still half an E in my backgammon case, the sniffer dog probably had a bad day.

I was summoned to police headquarters for questioning. I admitted that I had taken ecstasy on weekends for three months and was ordered to pay a fine of 3,600 Marks. The alternative was three months in jail. I borrowed the money.

Charlottenburg

Ben canceled my apartment share because Frank wanted to move in. I was pissed off, but what could I do? In the short term, I had to move back in with my parents, extremely unpleasant. A feeling of defeat. I often sat in my room, swung my colorful ceiling lamps back and forth, listened to Tom Waits, drank gin and tonic, and wrote poems or song lyrics. After three months, I moved to Berlin-Charlottenburg into a one-room apartment.

I had been given a book of Native American poems years ago. Each chapter had a picture symbol as a cover. I liked the sign of the firebird graphically very much. I had always wanted a tattoo, I had been carrying the thought around with me for three years. One morning I woke up still a bit woozy from the previous night and had 'Milk it' by Nirvana in my head, I woke up Sonja and we went to a tattoo studio.

I had this book with me, drank three beers and an hour later everything was done. It hurt. Anyone who says otherwise is either lying or into pain. A short time later I ended the relationship with Sonja, it led nowhere, it was nothing whole and nothing half. I wanted to be free again and go hunting.

Lotta

I was never a good student. I made up for my high school diploma in the second educational path. I only attended half of the three years and was on the verge of being expelled. Fortunately, the principal was a Social Democrat like me. I invited him to speak on education policy at an SPD summer party. He felt honored and a positive side effect was that I was not expelled from school. Sometimes they make it too easy, though.

Lotta was very much in need of harmony and family-oriented. I liked that, that's what I found in her. On top of that, a beautiful, very feminine figure. No wonder I stuck to her like gum wrappers for about seven years. We just couldn't get away from each other. Often briefly separated, then passion intervened and she had moved back in with me. That was one of her favorite things – moving. I remember: At the very beginning, in 1995, I was sitting on my mattress in my apartment, watching Star Trek, and Lotta was bringing things of hers. I guess I had said the night before that was okay ... but that her entire family shows up with a fleet of cars, she paints the bathroom pink, hangs pictures of abstractly painted women on my walls and I need a machete to fight my way to the toilet through all the new plants ... nooooo, nobody told me that before. Well, maybe I'm exaggerating a bit, but it's about right.

It was a great time, one of the best of my life. And like in an Italian opera, it crackled violently and regularly. The staircase was a great audience. She Scorpio, I Leo - oh shit!

Lotta had a beautiful classical singing voice, I admired that. We often went to karaoke parties with friends. At my brother-in-law's pool café, I was able to convince her to sing 'Ave Maria' at a Christmas party. It was great and I was proud of her.

She surprised me once when I came home from the office in a bad mood. There were rose petals spread in the apartment, candles everywhere and she was lying on the bed in suspenders. Wow, that was sexy, she loved me very much. It was too much for me at that moment, I came out of the office and I wasn't even really there yet, once again I hurt her feelings. I should have jumped on her. What did I do? ... I was insecure and my mind was somewhere else.

It was also good that Lotta talked all the time, because except for the occasional agitated, sometimes manic talk about politics and social justice in the world, I'm actually rather restrained verbally, so mostly, sometimes ... okay, once in a while. It started with, »When I woke up this morning,« and ended hours later with, »So, here I am and you didn't call me today.« If there was a soccer game on TV, it was a little annoying, but otherwise perfectly okay. I still think she started the vacuum cleaner during a game just to annoy me. Every half a year we talk on the phone and I know exactly what I have to do before-hand: go to the bathroom, eat something and chill at least two beers. Only then do I press the green phone button. I miss her sometimes and think of our time together. I also realize that today everything is different and only the memory remains. Nevertheless, I would like to know from time to time how she is doing and what she is up to. However, I can no longer imagine something like a friendship with her.

And my goodness, she had to endure a lot. When I think back to my soccer fanatic Hertha BSC Berlin days at the end of the nineties, she put up with it all. I could call her from anywhere at night - I didn't know where I was most of the time myself - and she would pick me up, no matter what manic excesses had gotten me into again. She loved me and I acted like a complete idiot most of the time, I loved her too. She called me 'rabbit'. We often watched the comedy series *Home Improvement*, I think that's why she called me that. Jill also called Tim like this in the german synchronization and somehow I often made a fool of myself. I could rarely really show her my affection, but the sex was phenomenal.

Signs of my psychological problems were already there when I was with Lotta. I remember that after an argument, I cut myself several times in the arm with a knife. Why I did that, I don't know. Actually, it's more common with borderliners.

Nowadays she is detached and cold, at least towards me. I don't think we have anything in common except our past. Her warm-heartedness at the time and a certain retro-50s fluffiness can only be read sporadically from some posts on Facebook. She extremely emphasizes her attitude: I can do everything myself and don't need any male dumbass. I think I have caused her a not inconsiderable amount of damage through our love affair, and that was certainly never my intention.

Her biological father came from the former Yugoslavia. I think this contributed to Lotta's increased sense of family - how shall I say? Maybe it was a positive dynamic from the uncertainty of her genetic origins. Just the other day her grandma passed away, so that must have taken a terrible toll on her. Her brother is also hugely important to her, a great guy, mathematically gifted, heavy metal guitarist and a self-contained person, I've always liked him.

Lotta's passion was and is cooking. I had a craving for fried potatoes one day and tried my hand at cooking. It went wrong and in despair I called Lotta. From then on, Sunday became our cooking day. For two to three hours we cooked, meaning she did, and I chopped and took notes on everything. Then we treated ourselves to a bottle of red wine with dinner and watched a movie. I enjoyed that a lot.

Lotta will hate me for this, but I can't help myself:

I learned that she used to cook spaghetti for some friends. She had used 8 oz of butter to prepare the pasta. When asked, she explained that there were no smaller portions to buy in the supermarket. They dutifully ate up and praised her, delicious. She now has her own catering service, which must be doing well.

I don't really remember how I met Lotta, I think it was on a bus on the way home from a party. We went to my place and she stayed the night. We made out, her skin was white and soft and smelled good.

When Lotta has an orgasm, she gets red marks on her face and she grins a little strangely.

I had stolen Lotta from a buddy, but she was as much involved in that as I was. Consequently, he hated me and, as I learned at the time, he threatened to hurt me very badly with a manslayer. Understandably, he was really pissed off. It quickly put things into perspective, he found his soul mate and is still with her today. We even became friends. Even as kids we had played field hockey together, but unfortunately today we have no contact anymore. There is hardly anyone from the old clique who still frequents *Club A18*.

Sex was very important to Lotta. Annoyed I was to the 1998 World Cup, because she constantly arrived with her sexual desire, without satisfaction she was obnoxious. Even while I was sleeping, she sometimes fiddled with me. I got tired of it and nailed her five or six times in one day so that she finally gave it a rest.

- short break for applause -

I even used dirty words - she wanted to try that. My hip bones, which she found strangely attractive, were blue the next day and my penis suffered a bruise. I had really given it my all, could hardly walk, but I could

79

at least watch the then World Cup peacefully - for a week. For sleeping we had a loft bed, it was only insufficiently fixed to the wall. When Lotta and I had fun, the bed banged rhythmically against the wall.

 The climax of her quite existing self-passion culminated in the fact that she attached a plaster cast of her breasts to the living room wall. It would never occur to me to put my penis or butt on display in the apartment for decoration, although ... eeh no. But never mind, I had some quirks at the time too. I don't want to write badly about Lotta, at least I try to restrain myself.

Southern men, for example from Turkey or the Arab world, had taken a fancy to her. I think she was curious about the culture and cuisine from those countries. I was told that she had some bad experiences after me. What attracts her today, I don't know. However, Lotta overly emphasizes that she is now a grown woman and that I was also just an experience for her. However, she also once remarked that I had spoiled her for manhood. She used to say, »I love you to the moon and back.« She liked Janosch's children's stories, especially the Tiger Duck.

Before I met Lotta, I had really let loose. I had things going on with a lot of women, almost every weekend, and my drug days were also before Lotta. She managed to make me feel happy in calmer waters, I had fallen in love. She still couldn't cope with my remaining wildness sometimes. I had interests in so many things that occasionally I simply forgot to show her my affection.

One beautiful winter day we went for a walk at the Wannsee lake, the snow provided wintry calm. We were once again on the verge of ending our relationship, yet this day was beautiful. In the end, we did not break up. In the restaurant *Loretta* at the Wannsee we talked it out. At that time I also had an appointment with a neurologist and he diagnosed depression. But it didn't bother me any further. Lotta had sent me to this examination because of my mood swings.

From time to time we visited a relative of her family, he must have been around 70 and was a painter, an artist. He drank a lot of wine and his studio impressed me. He had the ability to put moods and especially the character of people and a rather strange romanticism on canvas. I felt very much at home there.

My 20s were a really cool time and I spent most of them with Lotta. No matter how bitter she is about it today, I enjoyed them.

Lotta and I came back from a visit to her relatives in Essen. Somehow she was rattled and I had to drive the car on the way back, about six hours. I'm night blind and had to concentrate a lot. That was at Christmas time. In the evening we were finally back in Berlin at her parents' home. Still completely exhausted, I managed a slapstick interlude. I got up from the sofa, my head banged against the candlestick above the table, in shock I knocked over a floor lamp, which in turn crashed into the Christmas tree. The Christmas tree toppled over and the chaos was perfect. In my defense, I have to say that the whole house was cluttered with odds and ends, I had no choice but to bring the elephant-in-a-china-shop act. Fortunately, everyone had to laugh, no one was angry with me.

In July 2002 Lotta and I flew together on vacation, again Naxos. I think it was one of her first vacations in a European country. We had rented a nice little apartment at the *Maragas campground* for three weeks. I was looking forward to showing her my favorite place in the world. Lotta was a little nervous, but that quickly dissipated once we were on the ferry from Athens to Naxos. Salty wind and waves breaking on the ship.

After a few days, we sat at the camping bar in the evening and despite very warm weather, I felt shivery. It didn't feel good, something was wrong. Back at the apartment we took a fever, 102 degrees. Over the next few hours I shivered all over and my temperature rose to 109 degrees, I had a bad cough and I became frightened. Lotta made me ice-cold full-body wraps from bed sheets, but it didn't work anymore. I had to rush to the hospital, it was getting too dangerous. We went back to the camping bar to get help and I drank as much water as I could.

Normally, I like the Greek easy going: »If not today, then tomorrow, maybe.« In this situation, this attitude was completely out of place. The staff called a cab, but when nothing happened even after an hour, I yelled at the people:

»I'm fuckin' dying here, get a fuckin' taxi, NOW!«

After an hour and a half and three liters of water later, I was finally on my way to the hospital. The cab driver seemed to have all the time in the world and drove slow as fuck. During the day, when there are many people in Naxos town, they race like crazy through the area to pick up as many customers as possible. All that water brought the fever back down to 103 degrees upon arrival at the hospital. Pneumonia was diagnosed, one to two weeks of antibiotics.

July 28 was my birthday. Well great, drink orange juice and cigarettes only puff. Lotta had lit 30 tea lights on the terrace and it turned out to be a nice evening after all. Out of three weeks of vacation, I was ultimately down for only one week.

We took a trip to explore the island. I rented a scooter, Lotta a quad, those four-wheeled bumper cars. It was a beautiful day, we visited the small villages and enjoyed the Greek hospitality. The highlight was a visit to the church, I literally froze in humility before the beauty of this cathedral.

Lotta fell in love with the little alleys in the harbor district, especially the stores. Almost every evening she wanted to go shopping and I had to go with her, she bought and bought and I lugged all the stuff. But she also bought me a really fancy designer shirt, it had dice, pinup girls, aces of spades, Cadillacs and bubbly Champagne glasses on it. It was so ugly it was cool again. It's in Massachusetts somewhere now, I gave it to an old disheveled bartender later in my life who really liked that shirt, his name was Richy, I don't think he's alive today.

I asked Lotta what she thought about our vacation in retrospect. She thought Greece was just beautiful, but it was a difficult vacation. She didn't perceive it as a couple's vacation. Interpersonally, the vacation was a disaster, the whole relationship was a disaster in her opinion in this respect. She says she was always struggling to be seen and noticed by me. On vacation at a campsite in Greece you meet a lot of interesting people, of course I savored that, Lotta I also had at home day and night.

»**Love has nothing to do with how good or bad a relationship is.**«

I could never place this sentence of hers. Love always comes first for me, relationship problems are always there , but as long as love is there, everything is fine with me. It makes me think, I see a pattern. I've always been loved, but the in-between stuff has usually been a problem, where I end up again with not being able to open up. Clearly, I am a mess and anything but a sensible person, various doctors can attest to that.

The worst-case scenario occurs when two ex-girlfriends happen to meet for a chat, which is what happened at *Club A18*, my temporary exes Lotta and Gina. I should have run away right away, but couldn't, it was too exciting. They laughed conspicuously a lot, I already guessed what about: Sex, what else. They also made friends, there's no way out, you've lost anyway.

I was very shocked when Ralf died and all Lotta said was, »That was obvious, he lived unhealthily.« Even if it is the truth, you don't say something like that when you are mourning a dear friend. I was shocked and I realized once again that her character does not conform to mine.

Germerica

From 9:00 a.m. to 2:00 p.m. I studied at the Berlin Mediadesign Academy, then I worked until 8:00 p.m. on the sinking ship real estate company. Gerhard Schröder became chancellor in 1998 and he actually closed some tax loopholes. Just sucked for the company, but correct. I lived in a nice two-room apartment in Berlin-Wannsee. A short-lived relationship was over and Lotta was here and there. Any attempts to separate us always failed because of our passion for each other. I wouldn't say love-hate, more something like not with and not without each other.

My cat and I usually sat at the PC in the evening. I was often in an American chat room where users could even upload pictures in the page frame. Please note that it was 2002 and therefore revolutionary. Today it is hard to imagine, but intercontinental conversation on the net was new. It was the time of Yahoo messenger with video function. I struck up a conversation with Melonie. Like a lot of Americans, Melonie claimed that she was partly of Native American descent, apparently that's part of the cool tone over there.

The time difference between Berlin and Massachusetts is six hours. For three months I spent the nights chatting with Melonie. As a result, I was sometimes absent from class. But as is often the case, I didn't have to make much of an effort to get my diploma, high school diploma, business degree, or anything else. Such things were rather incidental, the main thing was that I had something to do.

Melonie made me curious, she was different. She had a son, at 19 she had had him, Michael. I got more and more the feeling that I belonged there. I looked at photos and thought, »Yes, this is your job!« One night I called her for the first time and there it was again, the stuttering under emotional stress, this time in English, she thought it was cute. She liked it when I said »Water« with a hard T.

Editor's note: No man wants to be cute.

I knew right away that it wasn't going to be an easy number, a lot to do. At that time I was still indestructible, I simply breathed in the world. No fear, no worries, nothing was impossible, but the chaos in my head was omnipresent. I always had continuous fire in my head.

America

In 2003, I gave up a vacation in Greece and jumped across the pond for four weeks to see Melonie. I could afford it, I had previously won at soccer betting. On the airport shuttle bus, everyone was babbling gum. I may have been manic, but the world was my oyster. Nothing could stop me, I was free, severely confused but free. Some people at the time thought I was running away from my problems, I didn't think so. I followed my heart, rationality was never my thing. Well, they were a little bit right. In retrospect, I think I had hope that a new love would make everything better. I am somehow always lonely in my own way. I'm sure most people can relate to that.

Boston, Logan Airport. I came out of the frosted glass doors and there she was already ... wow ... everything done right. This constant »Welcome to America« from all sides was annoying, I first put in 'Dickes B' by the Berlin Band Seeed on the way to Westfield in 'Uncle Bob's new truck' to feel safer. But our common song later became 'Blurry' by Puddle of Mudd.

A typical American small town, just like you know it from the movies. Some wooden houses even had a white picket fence, the streets were patchwork, the power lines above ground. Then the most fucked up house on the street was the one where Melonie, Michael and some family members lived. Her two brothers were the welcoming committee, could have been that I was some kind of perverted German internet freak. I know what you are thinking. No, I'm not.

The five-room apartment was the top floor of the house. Michael, then five years old, came running up the outside stairs with big, expectant eyes. So now I was to be a good surrogate father. The first thing he insisted on was that I read to him from a dinosaur book. I wasn't very good, very slow and nervous, but he still liked it and looked at me with a look I'll never forget, he looked at me like I was a savior or something. I realized that he was longing for something, very longing.

I was shocked at the condition of the apartment, what a dump. The bathroom had an open wall, I could practically bathe outside and wave to the neighbors. The clothes dryer was held together with the help of a chair and a hammer. I spent three weeks making our floor a little more livable, it was completely cluttered. There wasn't even a vacuum cleaner, but I had guessed something like that, I was okay with it.

On the very first evening we went to *Froggies*, a country pub with bright neon lights, on Fridays there was karaoke. There we sat across from each other, Melonie and I, and could first take a deep breath, having arrived. I was overwhelmed by all the new impressions in such a short time. I think I stared at her rather strangely that night, in a good way.

I wasn't familiar with the bar rules in America, the tip is just left open on the counter and when it's closing time, they just take your beer away. Of course that didn't work for me and I was already involved in a fight, they didn't really like me, I was just too European. Melonie dragged me out of the bar and loaded me into the car. I asked her later in bed, »I'd like to kiss you, is that okay?« It was okay. Sex ensued and I was a bit puzzled, normally women do moan during orgasm. With her, I was confronted with whiny sounds. Her favorite line after sex was always, »Damn, this gun was loaded!« And she was aggressive in bed, my goodness, was she aggressive. Sex had to be her life. I didn't mind it at first. There was a whole drawer of sex toys next to the bed. I always catch women who like to be on top, but maybe that's generally the case, I don't know.

New York City

Of course I wanted to see New York City, only a four-hour drive from Westfield. Melonie was still freshly in love with me and I managed to persuade her to go. That wasn't so easy, she was a bit of a country bumpkin and didn't like big cities.

It was summer and near the coast on the way to New York, in the car, I smelled sea air. We were at the crest of the Williamsburg Bridge when the car gave up the ghost. Luck of the draw, we were able to roll down the rest of the bridge and the momentum was still enough to turn into a side street. Melonie was having a crisis. She stayed with the car and I ran to organize a tow truck. Big city – my thing. It was already early evening. After two hours I found a garage, they in turn called a tow truck and together we drove back to Melonie and collected her. The repair would take until the next morning. He dropped us off at a hotel that was probably the cheapest in the area. However, we couldn't check into our room until 10:00 p.m., an hourly hotel for 150 $ a night.

First rest in a small café, a Coke and two small Guinness, made 22 $, we went then rather. At the gas station across from the hotel we got chips, sandwiches, a six-pack of Becks beer and cigarettes, 38 $. We sat down on a bench in front of the hotel and witnessed a cab driver smash the windows of the car in front of him and beat up the driver.

It got dark and a black guy with gold teeth and a yellow and white snake around his neck came by and offered us drugs. We declined with thanks, Melonie always had her own weed with her. It started to rain, but then we could finally move into our room. The air conditioning was set very cold. Melonie didn't mind, she had a natural protection against the cold, and cuddling and screwing kept me warm.

Michael had graduation at school the next day, was probably important. I saw Melonie crying for the first time, because she was afraid she couldn't be there because of the broken car. The next morning we took a cab to the garage, the repair cost 700 $. Around 1000 $ we had spent in less than 24 hours in New York City and I saw almost nothing of the city.

We still made it to Michael's graduation. The only time I saw Melonie crying again was when she slipped on spaghetti in the kitchen that Michael had spilled earlier. She is a very strong woman who very rarely shows weakness.

The marriage proposal

For the marriage proposal, I asked her roommate Doris to send me a ring from Melonie by mail to Berlin, so that the size would be right. She had 64 and I had wedding rings made, silver and plain.

I then flew over for the second time and wanted to ask her the question of all questions. I talked to her mother, who was the owner of the house and lived on the first floor, and asked her to cook a delicious dinner, I got a bottle of champagne.

We went to *Froggies* for karaoke. My sister was pregnant for the first time at the time. The plan was for Melonie's mom to call *Froggies* and tell Melonie that there was trouble with my sister Luisa and her pregnancy and that I needed to call my family urgently.

Once home a romantic dinner was served, I got down on one knee and asked her to marry me. She said »Yes.« Apparently she liked me. After two weeks I had to go back to Germany.

I had sent Melonie money from Berlin for a new car and a book plus CD-ROM English-German. She was interested in words like *dick* or *fucking*. To this day she doesn't know what *Yes* and *No* or *Salt* and *Pepper* mean in German. Weak performance. If I had a Spanish girlfriend, I would of course learn Spanish immediately.

Continental drift

For four months I prepared everything to emigrate for good: Forms, embassy, doctors, apartment and a farewell party at *Club A18*.

And some things of the preparation were even painful, at 32 I had myself circumcised, there were problems during sex. That was extremely uncomfortable, I was so nervous with fear that they had to inject me with something as I was lying on the operating table shaking. I assume it was morphine. What followed was five weeks of evening bathtub sessions with chamomile extract, sex-free dreams, and a ban on Melonie showing pictures in chat. Well, she often sent me sexy pictures of herself. Inconvenient in this situation, I had to try to think of soccer results. That was frustrating, Hertha BSC played really crappy at that time.

Then the time had come. All my friends and family said goodbye to me at Berlin-Tegel airport, many tears flowed. Lotta gave me a book, in which she had stuck souvenir photos of us and decorated it with lyrics from Element of Crime. But she was actually angry with me. I just took off like that, I think that thwarted her plans a bit. By the time I got to Melonie's house, I was completely wiped out. I realized that this was going to be a different life now.

A big problem was my residence and work permit. It was an enormous amount of bureaucracy. After all, I was an import and we had to get married in order for me to stay. Melonie hated having to fill out forms, she had virtually no understanding of why I couldn't handle it on my own. But my English was just too bad for officialese. Everything cost a lot of money and effort.

Six weeks after my re-arrival in Massachusetts, my four boxes also arrived by ship. I drove the 91 miles with Melonie's father, Francis, to Boston Harbor to pick up my luggage. I was uncomfortable sitting in the car with my father-in-law for so long. I made an effort to lighten the mood a bit with music, but Francis was cool and we spent a pleasant man's day together after all. He took me out for a lobster dinner at *Red Lobster* in Boston Harbor. I unfortunately had to tell him that I don't like fish, that irritated him, before that I told him that I like to cook.

There was this one moment, Melonie and I were at *Davio's*, a bar around the corner. Melonie rarely and reluctantly went out unless it was to karaoke, where she could be the center of attention, that was typical of her. Anyway, we sat there and I looked at her and *bam*! I was head over heels in love, it tingled.

In Westfield, it was the custom that when women went to a club without wanting to pay admission, all they had to do was pull up their outerwear at the entrance. I was out by myself and I struck up a conversation with two of these thrifty gals. After a fun evening, I then came home around 2:00 a.m.. I just flirted a bit, nothing more had happened. Melonie was sitting on our bed looking at me pretty pissed off. »Did you have fun tonight?« I said yes, was nice. I don't know how, but she knew. Of course I denied everything, stupidly the phone rang then and two giggling women were on the line. She was so pissed off. How the girls got our phone number was beyond me. I could not possibly have been so stupid.

Grandiose was also my performance when I peed against a wall after a bar visit and was arrested. I relieved myself at the police station of all places from the dullsville and the outside camera caught me doing it. I spent a few hours in a cell. Fucking up things – I´m good at.

What I didn't know was that there are so-called jack-and-jill parties for couples who want to get married, a joint bachelor party, if you will. We went on stage, we were asked questions, and we had to endure games. Of course, the night before our wedding, I partied hard again alone with my new friends and Melonie's two brothers.

A general problem was that things get around very quickly in a small town, I had to get used to that. Melonie always knew about everything, it didn't look good for my usual lifestyle.

My parents hadn't seen me for two months and flew over to the US for the wedding. I will never forget the look on my mother's face when she fell around my neck full of love at the airport. It makes my eyes go pee-pee when I remember that.

After we arrived at my new home, my mom was speechless, it was still a dump. When it comes to cleanliness, she is very meticulous. She immediately started inspecting everything, cleaning and helping prepare for the wedding ceremony. She has a Scottish accent, as a teenager she had lived there for several years. My father seemed a bit helpless, not really fluent in english.

Every time I flew across the pond and arrived in Massachusetts, I got sick first, and so did my parents. The tap water tasted like chemicals and rust. Melonie always got angry when I criticized something about America. I can understand that, but it was a fact, and we Germans are known for criticizing everything - with a Berlin snout anyway. But when Melonie packed a piece of meat in a plastic foil on Styrofoam to defrost in the microwave, I just had to say something, I couldn't help it.

Melonie always turned up the air conditioning full blast. Even when I had a painful ear infection, she insisted on keeping the cool breeze. I was angry and she was annoyed because she had to drive me to the hospital at night. Character-wise, I couldn't relate. If she had been miserable, I would have done anything to make her feel better.

The wedding

I insisted on a church wedding, at least that I could enforce. I had already taken her name and changed the continent. In addition, I was allowed to choose the song for the dance at the wedding ceremony, my choice fell on Procol Harum's 'A whiter shade of pale'. Melonie and I had a conversation with the priest beforehand, it was about the course of the ceremony. The fact that I took Melonie's last name was suspicious to her. I made it clear to her that I did not attach much importance to it.

With her brother Stan, I went for a quick drive right before the wedding to get a bow tie for my wedding outfit. He asked me in the car, »How does it feel to only fuck one pussy for the rest of your life?« I didn't answer, I mean he called his sister pussy, hello?

Melanie's mom tailored the wedding dress for her. She has many talents, I must say. Her turkey for Thanksgiving was a blast. I was grateful that she organized the main part of the wedding. I'm pretty sure she has some kind of thing going on. It has to be something sexual. She always has lovers about 20 years younger. She's got something going on.

Melonie's dress had a shimmery pearl effect, she also made a beaded wreath for her hair, a bit hippie style. Aunt Anni was commissioned by me to take photos. Unfortunately, she did not succeed very well, that was annoying.

In the church I felt very different, as if I were in a surreal movie, very strange. I stood at the altar and Melanie's father led her forward to the music. I had tears in my eyes, as did my parents. My nose was running and I tried to signal to my best man, Stan, that I needed a tissue. He didn't have one with him, so I sniffled to myself. I hope in the excitement no one noticed.

Not only Melonie and I were asked about our love at the ceremony, Michael was too. All three of us said »I do«.

I was full of beans and wanted to build us a future. After the wedding ceremony we went to an open-air restaurant in a wooded area, lots of steaks and burgers. We danced, first Melonie and I, then Father Francis high-fived and finally my mother danced with me. For this dance I chose the theme from the movie *Leolo*.

I was the happiest person that day.

It's customary for the bride and groom to slap the wedding cake in each other's faces. I think I did this a little too intensely, but was not a problem. After a nice speech by Stan, everyone changed into jeans and t-shirts, it was very hot, over 90 degrees. I didn't do this on this special day, but my bride felt a little cramped in her dress. It was a great party. I didn't know then that the circumstances and the illness would shatter my dreams.

The honeymoon was a long weekend at a hotel in a neighboring town, the room had a jacuzzi, but otherwise it was a shabby flophouse.

Mr. & Mrs.

So Melonie and I were now newlyweds. We went to a chat website party at a hotel. It was interesting to meet the people from the Internet. Melonie liked to say, »This is my husband.« Unfortunately, the party only went on until just after midnight. So-called room parties followed, and that's when things really got going. A wet towel sealed the door slit so no one outside could smell that there was smoking in the room. In our suite, there were about ten of us partying.

Two women, Sophia and Doreen, were also there, a lesbian couple. Doreen was the dominant part in the relationship. We were all in a good mood and somehow it came about that Doreen and I had some kind of wrestling on the bed. I don't know why I got involved, she had challenged me, I couldn't possibly have this on my back.

My newlywed wife was really pissed and she let me feel it the next day. On the drive home, we barely spoke a word to each other. When we got home, she hissed, »I want the divorce.« I realized that I had really screwed up and could only apologize. As an argument, I said that Doreen was a lesbian and we were just fooling around. Unfortunately, this argumentation remained ineffective. Melonie had something against excuses and apologies in principle. I wasn't very good at it either. For two weeks I was good and then it went again, she had forgiven me.

I was still in contact with Sophia and Doreen for a long time, they now lived in Florida. Doreen tragically had some kind of infection, something in her brain, I don't know the details. She had to learn to speak again. This strong woman was only a shadow of her former self. A year ago she passed away, I was very sad. R.I.P. Doreen. Sophia unfortunately also passed away the other day, may the good Lord take care of her good soul. Greetings upwards.

Melonie got jealous if I even looked at another woman from the car. She would say something like, »Do you see something you like?« If I wanted to listen to Rammstein or Oasis in the car, that was a problem. Melonie loved Fiona Apple and other 'strong women' and always sang along very loudly. It was pure torture for me and it made her very unattractive when I looked over at her like that.

Once, by accident, the wedding ring slipped off Melonie's finger into the trash, of all things, and she said, »Oh, that's a bad omen.« I lost my ring on the way home from work, it fell out of my pocket while I was riding my bike. Employees weren't allowed to wear rings while making pizza.

We had agreed in advance on Yahoo that I could go out once a week, with her or without her. I made it clear to her that I am a night person and need social contact like the air I breathe. When I was finally on the scene, I was promptly forbidden to do so. And when I did get my way and was out for two or three hours on the weekend, the result was that the mood was lousy until at least Wednesday, unless we had sex in between. Then it was okay, then she had her confirmation. She seemed anything but insecure, but I suspect deep down she was. When I went out alone, she would always say to me, with her finger raised, »Stay out of trouble.« She had noticed pretty quickly that I kind of attracted trouble, even though I wasn't actually doing anything bad.

The style of dancing in the USA is very different from what we do in Europe. The Yanks always act as if they are having sex on the dance floor.

Melonie would often say »You know, Nino?« because it rhymed and »I don't know.« The latter sounded something like: »Indunno.« My inadequate English skills annoyed her, and again, I didn't like that at all. A little more consideration would have been nice. I decided to speak only German for a day to make her understand how it was for me. She got angry and I broke off the experiment early to save my ass.

When women gripe, they call it communication. When men do it, it's an argument.

Melonie got really upset when I just walked away during an argument, this usually happened when she was arguing with me but I wasn't arguing with her.

She always counted threateningly from one to three when our son disobeyed, it worked. Once even with me, how embarrassing.

I often retreated to our small corner room. The windows were open in the summer and I drank my beer there in the evening. Not far away were railroad tracks, I liked the sound of the passing trains at night.

Her ex, Michael's producer, is probably an asshole, he beat her and dragged her out of a bar by her hair, for example, she told me. Vodka was his breakfast, so a real champ. She got hurt a lot and I had to take the heat for it. As soon as I got anywhere near his behavior, Melonie snapped, or at least made me feel very clearly that she was upset. How could I help it that this jerk had treated her so badly in the past?

I would have taken my problems with me, Lotta wrote me in an email. Even my problems had problems, but we loved each other and that was important. In retrospect, I think she loved the idea or the idea of me, but not me.

The relationships with Nicola, Lotta and Melonie had two things in common: all three claimed to be pregnant. They were not pregnant and lied to me to find out how I would react. I flipped out in anger each time. How could they be so hardened to my feelings? There is nothing more important in a man's life than fathering a child. You don't play with feelings like that. Another thing Lotta and Melonie had in common was that they both tried to make money with phone sex, but then broke off disappointed. I suppose they had hoped for more from it,maybe nice men who felt like having an erotic conversation and not perverted drunken assholes they had to listen to while they jerked off.

Melanie's friend Lisa came to visit for the weekend and in the evening we went to *Froggies* again and partied hard. My favorite song that I always performed was Oasis' 'Champagne Supernova', I was pretty good at that.

Back home, the two wanted to have a sexy photo session. Me with two naked women who made out with each other on the bed, the camera at the ready. Sometimes the good Lord has meant well with me.

The two were up quite early the next morning and already smoking pot again. Melonie's humor was cheeky and black. She woke me up frantically, said she had ordered pizza and I had to leave quickly to pick her up. Pants on, stumbled down the outside stairs, into the car and off to our regular pizzeria, *Pasqualis*. Once there, an employee gave me a strange grin.

»Aren't you Nino, the husband of Melonie?«
»Ehh, yes.«
»You're from Germany, right?«
»I am, why?«
»Nothing, you're all set, Sir. Two Pizza Peperoni.«

She turned briefly to the open kitchen and the kitchen crew started grinning as well. Slightly confused, I headed back home. Aunt Anni was sitting in front of the door on the first floor and looked at me just as overly friendly.

While my two stoners were eating their pizzas, I went into the bathroom and looked in the mirror. My sweetheart had painted a Hitler moustache on me while I slept and on my forehead was written 'Dork'.

She was of the opinion that my little lower lip beard should be a little higher, under my "big German nose", as she always said. Well, it's not thaaaaat big.

As we were driving in the car, we were pulled over by a cop. Melonie rolled down the window and said, »I'll take a double cheeseburger, small fries and a Coke.« The cop couldn't manage to stay serious and let us continue our way.

You surely know those greeting cards that you open and a music sounds. Melonie took the thing out and stuck it on Michael's back, the poor guy walked around all day wondering why some movements always sounded a melody. Greeting cards are an integral part of holidays in America, of even the most unimpoertant holidays in america.

The summerwind

My dream was always to live by the sea, good for the soul, such a vast, powerful ocean. Melonie and I planned to move, out of the small town. I had only one condition: the sea. We discussed that a lot. For her, a good school for Michael was an absolute priority. I agreed, but it couldn't be that there wasn't a single good school on the entire east coast of the USA.

There was a rocker bar that I liked. I was sitting at the bar and a biker sat down next to me. He noticed my accent and asked where I was from. I said, »I'm from Germany.« His reply was, »Oh yeah, I hate niggers, too.« Horrified, I ordered another beer.

Once again, I proved my talent for clumsiness. I hadn't yet gotten used to the door handles in America, which only have this round knob. In the evening I came home and automatically grabbed a normal european door handle and elegantly banged my head against the door. Fortunately, no one saw that.

It was family function day. Sometimes the entire family got together, which must have been something like 70 people. These meetings took place either in Stanley Park or at a family's house in the backyard. I never really felt like it, petty banter and appallingly tasteless burgers.

On days like that, I would cook something delicious, but retreat to our small, four-square-meter corner room and listen to german music. I thought of beautiful winter days with my family in ski resorts in Austria or Switzerland and felt homesick. I downloaded German movies and series from the Internet to make my homesickness more bearable or maybe even intensify it.

Nowhere in Westfield was there an outdoor café or beer garden, nothing where people could gather in the summer. That was only possible privately in your own backyard.

In America, it's a little disconcerting that many people are too lazy to walk. The walk to my workplace at the pizzeria was about ten minutes, with family members constantly asking me if they should drive me there. Very friendly in itself, but I preferred to walk. My wife took the car across the street to the video store, just across the street. She also preferred to look for a parking space in the huge parking lot in front of Walmart for 15 minutes rather than having to park too far away from the entrance.

It is remarkable that in supermarkets also sometimes hard rock music is played. I stood at the checkout, behind an 80-year-old woman, and 'Chop Suey' by System of a Down was played as background music, cool. Unthinkable in Germany.

Forced to be a househusband for a year, I also became more and more depressed due to the situation. My parents supported me financially, but still it is hard for any man to be kept. I cleaned, cooked and took care of son-man as best I could. But I was also preoccupied with myself and not always one hundred percent on task. I felt inferior, I was not well.

After a while, Melonie actually only came home from work frustrated, she hated her job. No »Hi Honey«, no kiss, no touch ... nothing. She sat down at her computer, rolled a joint and enjoyed the attention of her chat admirers. This was poison for our relationship, I was not happy about it.

I had gone for the cheap beer brand Pabst Blue Ribbon, which was really, really bad. Melonie thinks beer is evil and cannabis is a godsend. Smoking pot is not my thing, I always just get dumb as untoasted white bread, tired, get the munchies, my circulation fails or I don't know if I'm about to pee or not. Something spiritual or mentally interesting doesn't happen. When smoking pot, my sweetheart used tweezers to smoke even the last bit of the joint.

Basically, she had the attention span of a fruit fly on LSD.

Often she had back or neck pain. I should then always take a suitable pressure device and press it against her pain point with great force for one or two minutes, and when I let go, a feeling of relaxation would follow.

Melonie is convinced of her spiritual powers. So one evening she held a pendulum in her fingers and claimed she could move it by the power of her thoughts. She demonstrated it. I took the pendulum and stapled it to the Styrofoam ceiling ... »Okay, try it now.« Of course she couldn't and got pissed off.

Her penchant for self-love reached its verbal peak when she said to me, »If I could, I would marry myself.«

Her sex addiction also became a problem for me. Almost every night when we weren't making love, she was masturbating next to me in bed. You can imagine how that made me feel ... humiliated. The pressure to please her became stronger and stronger and had the opposite effect, I withdrew more and more. I'm not the type who just wants to fuck. Small expressions of affection are very important to me, love must always be felt.

Michael had ADHD, which is attention deficit disorder. I never told Melonie that something like that could come from smoking pot during pregnancy, she would have lynched me. He just left everything, was almost impossible to get out of bed in the morning, and then the other extreme, hyperactivity, a whirlwind that could not be controlled. Teachers often called me to ask me to pick him up from school because he was disturbing the lessons. But Michael was a smart guy though, read Harry Potter and regularly beat me at the game Checkers. Unfortunately, he was very often out of control and when we gave him his medication, he was no longer himself, totally run down, a condition you could not bear as a parent.

At one very bad stage, he even threatened me with a kitchen knife, I did not get along with the boy at times. It took a very long time until he accepted me. I am also not the type to exude parental authority. At Christmas time, Melonie, Michael and I went out to get a Christmas tree. I have to admit, that's when slight father feelings came up in me, I had never done anything like that before. After all, I was teaching Michael to play soccer and ride a bike, that's what daddies do, right? It was also nice when I was told that Michael proudly said at school that he now had two daddies.

At this point I must praise Hertha BSC, the Berlin soccer team, I wrote an email and asked for autograph cards for Michael, they did immediately, free of charge.

Every night at bedtime, Michael would put his hands around my neck and his legs around my waist and I would swing back and forth on all fours and we would count the swings in German. In a year and a half we got to exactly 3,333. We called this ritual the 'Monkey'. Occasionally we played soccer inside, Melonie didn't like it at all and she was like, »Oh shit, now I have two kids, no playing inside, damnit.« She often complained that she always had to be the bad one when it came to raising children, but when I snapped once and gave Michael a telling off, she wasn't happy with that either, now that was too harsh again. In this regard, we rarely saw eye to eye on this.

In the middle of our king size bed, between our heads, was a clock radio and Melonie listened to the rock station all night. She said it calmed her down and helped her fall asleep. This was not the case with me and I had many sleepless nights. On top of that she had teeth grinding and snoring, most of the time I went into the living room completely unnerved and watched TV. Now she hated that again, she wanted to have me by her side at night. Every evening she got massages from me and when she fell asleep, I would sneak away.

When I finally got my work permit, I took a job at *Skypizza*, which was good for me. Sometimes it was 15-hour shifts. I felt fine when I came home from work completely knocked out and could snuggle up with my wife around midnight. I finally had a job and that was nice. Except for Aaron, I liked my co-workers, all cool. Aaron supported Bush, that just didn't work, plus he was very stupid and always called the young boss 'ma'am'.

When I was employed there, I thought about how I could show my love to Melonie. I then baked a heart-shaped pizza for her and with some ingredients I wrote 'I love you' on it. I didn't have much money, so I had to improvise.

After only a few weeks, my beloved demanded that I look for a second job or find a better-paying job. That was not fair. She wanted me to do everything. I was under a lot of pressure, most people get aggressive or something, it was different for me: a co-worker, Shannon, was pregnant, standing on the making line working on pizza dough. Brandon, a delivery driver, came in and asked her:

»Hey, Shannon, if I would have Sex with you, would that mean I would have Sex with two girls?«

I saw the horrified look on Shannon's face and couldn't stop laughing for two hours. I almost choked, all my stress bubbling out of me. I think I seemed a little crazy.

In a shop window I discovered a painting. The background was washed out pink. It depicted how a tadpole becomes a frog, circular, in a kind of life cycle. I knew Melonie would like it, that's just how my stoner chick was.

»This is totally me.« She was happy. At the same time, however, she complained that I only ever arrived with gifts or flowers when I messed up.

Sometimes I would just call her at the office and sing 'I just called to say I love you' to her. So I think I was already making an effort.

Sex sells

Melonie was anything but slim, which is nothing special in the States. She was also aware that there are a lot of men who find exactly that attractive. There are now a lot of portals, forums, chat rooms, singles exchanges and all sorts of other stuff, sometimes sick shit that I want nothing to do with. Every pot has its lid. I like it just round, I take that for granted.

An friend of ours recognized this niche early on and hosts special party events in hotels in Massachusetts. She has been doing this every three to four weeks for about 15 to 20 years now. She and her husband Jimmy make a lot of money doing it. Jimmy was a Canadian import and we hit it off. It wasn't until later that I found out they wanted to have communal sex with us.

So it happened that Melonie wanted to have her own sexy website, a member site. For 12.95 $, there was a photo set of 40 pictures and a video every ten days. I didn't mind and took on the project. We bought a new camera and a construction spotlight at *Homedepot*. I had completed the website, now I busied myself with making the pictures look good and edited them on the computer before putting them online. Melonie enjoyed being photographed and having her face on the web. The website was well received and we were making some money.

Breathe deeply for a sec

After one and a half years, I was officially allowed to leave the USA again. I had missed my family very much, missed the births of my two nephews. What if something bad happened and I couldn't be there? I flew to Berlin for two weeks and spent two more weeks with the family in Greece. My wife was pissed. How could I have left her alone? I think I had more than earned this vacation.

During my visit to Berlin there was a mega rock party at *Club A18*. How I had missed that, getting senselessly drunk and rocking out until the doctor comes, finally back in my on my turf.

I reflected on my situation while on vacation. In Berlin and in Greece I found some distance. To be honest, I had my freedom back and it felt good. I realized that it couldn't go on like this. I resolved to be stronger and do my thing.

Failed

My wife didn't like that at all. It took three weeks for Melonie to get fed up with my new assertiveness, turn to me at my desk and say, »I can't do this anymore.«

Oddly, our big bed had collapsed when I got back from Berlin. I found a Red Sox lighter and burst condoms while cleaning up. I approached her about it and she told me that a friend was visiting. Since she had about the same figure as Melonie, the bed had collapsed and they had just been playing around with the condoms. Who would believe it.

In the final phase of our marriage, when we were once again arguing, her mother approached us and asked us to list the things we loved about each other. Spontaneously I thought of: her humor, her looks and her quirk of always wanting to see everything positively. She liked my looks and all the information I had. She intentionally did not use the word intelligence because she was very proud of her spiritual intelligence and did not want to hide it under a bushel. She saw herself, as she said, several levels above me.

In the two weeks until my flight back to Berlin, we avoided each other as best we could. I went out in the evenings, drank too much and my heart was in a thousand pieces, I was completely at the end. All the strength, the love, the hope and the dreams ... all gone. My world collapsed. That was the most emotionally cruel moment in my life. I started stuttering again and couldn't comprehend it all. Everything was taken away from me, I was in ruins.

I'm pretty sure my wife talks bad about me to family and friends after the fact, that's how she is. She will do anything to make herself look good. This bothers me, I can't tell the other side of the coin, I can't do anything about a partially false image of me.

When I left, I left chaos in the apartment. I had given up cleaning for weeks, I didn't want to do it anymore. After all, the apartment was in better condition than I had found it.

Was it unfair of me not to be ready for this relationship? She wanted my help, I wanted hers and it almost worked out, actually we fit together quite well. I wasn't ready yet. Today I am happy to be with my family in Berlin.

She gave me as a parting gift a necklace pendant with some sacred figure, I don't know exactly who it was, some saint. She said it was a Guardian Angel to protect me. She had recognized that I had psychological problems. However, she was not willing to work on our relationship. She actually asked me if I could continue running the sex website from Berlin. Money-hungry bitch. Of course I didn't, I'm not completely stupid.

I had taken all my important and personal belongings with me when I moved to America, and when I left in a hurry, much had remained in the attic of the house. Upon inquiring with the family, I was told that everything was gone. That was sad, some things meant a lot to me.

The fact that I had failed abroad shook my self-confidence to the core. I had always thought I could do anything.

Institution and psychiatrist

Then in December 2005 I was taken to a closed institution for a few days, I was depressed, confused and aggressive, couldn't cope at all. They assumed that I could hurt myself, I was locked up. For the first time I really met lunatics and drug zombies. Instead of assigning individual rooms to these people and giving them special care, I spent the night in a hall with eight beds and barred windows. There was rioting and yelling all night. The nurses constantly came by and gave the patients injections or shit-egg pills. No fucking way to get some sleep.

Fortunately, after three days I was transferred to the normal psycho wing, a room in the first class became available. Everything else was occupied, lucky me, I'm a state insured patient.

The next few weeks were very lonely, they didn't know exactly what to do with me. I am an actor who always keeps up the facade as long as I can.

Then it was Christmas and the year before I had spent it with my wife and my stepson, a trigger, with me all dams broke, they had to sedate me. The rest was white, quiet snow outside the window and quite a drone.

A guy who had just sat next to me in the group and finally said something was dead the next morning. That was announced to us at breakfast. He had gone out and thrown himself out of the window at his ex-girlfriend's house. Love can do bad things.

Also unfortunate was a circa 50-year-old woman who always just sat in her chair, never said anything, and stared, just stared. That was very sad, she was lost.

And then this guy, tall and fat, half-bald, mad look, I suspected he would eat babies. I had to keep avoiding him as best I could. Why is it that people just like that are always so fixated on me? I seem to attract something like that, as if I of all people could help them. Many like to dump their problems on me, I must have such an charisma or way about me.

Then there was a young girl with borderline syndrome and an insurance salesman who had a severe drinking problem. I used to hang out with them in the smoking room. Most girls with borderline syndrome tend to seek validation through sex just to be able to feel anything. They often even seek intimacy with women when nothing else works. Which is absolutely okay, of course. However, that has just been my observation over the years. It doesn't have to be true. I was good at observing from an early age, I perceived the world very intensively in my own way.

Every person needs affection, even if it is only physical.

The entire ward 16 in the clinic was an over-excited bunch of borderline lesbians, very entertaining.

The first psychiatrist I went to, which was in 2005, stated in horror, »You're in a pitiful state.« A few months later, unfortunately, he died of colon cancer.

He prescribed me antidepressants. After a few weeks it helped somewhat. I lived provisionally in a basement room with my parents, nothing was mine. It became autumn and my condition worsened. Everything I had tried to build, a family, my own thing, it was shattered just like that, I was set back years. The strength to fight yourself out of such a low again is very difficult to muster and sustain.

I was on my way to my first psychotherapist. A slimy, self-absorbed, arrogant 'Dr. Psycho'. It was mid-morning and I was on the subway.

Gray and dreary, everything was unreal, a non-feeling, I was non-existent. I looked at the display board S3 to Charlottenburg and stood there for ten minutes, not knowing what it meant. That's how absent-minded you can be when you're severely depressed. Nothing makes sense, nothing in this world. Someone spoke to me, he spoke to me, but I couldn't perceive him, like a soundless little film.

The therapist's first question was, »Are you gay?« I asked him what made him think that. »You wear an earring." I had to explain to him that many men wear an earring and only with the right ear could one possibly conclude that the person was gay. After half an hour, I realized that he was in no way meeting the professional requirements of a therapist.

Dr. Psycho tried to salvage something, unfortunately after four, maybe five sessions he couldn't establish any kind of access to me and I also knew that I could never open up to that type of person. It rarely happens to me that I can't get along with someone, this time it was like that. By the way, I expect answers from psychotherapists and not this attitude - »Let him talk, he'll figure it out himself.« The phrase »What are YOU thinking?« is one I hate.

I moved to the seventh floor of a high-rise building in Berlin-Ze-hlendorf, the hallways were white and cold, I probably would have killed myself there at some point, I had never felt so alone before. I felt as if I had also been deported by my family.

When I didn't show up for a therapy session and Dr. Psycho called my parents and told them he wasn't guaranteeing anything anymore, they called the fire department and they broke down my apartment door. I had been unresponsive to calls, asleep, and had these earplugs in my ears, so didn't hear anything. Almost one hundred percent of depressed people are not useful in the morning, they are nocturnal. So where does a shrink get the idea that a patient is on his doorstep at nine o'clock in the morning in the sticks and open to anything? I screamed with rage, feeling even shabbier in my already shabby world. This apartment was a cell for me, I was not alive and dead sad.

I looked for a new job, any job. I became a pizza driver at an Italian restaurant on Kurfürstendamm. Dirty place, dirty owner, he lived in his store. Only poor people from Romania worked in the kitchen. The boss turned over every cent three times, but only out of greed for money. It was interesting that he was involved with the mafia, somehow I have always had a penchant for crooks. I'm just not good at it, probably because I like people on principle. I mostly supplied brothels in Berlin-Charlottenburg, his ancient grandma, or shady guys playing poker in back rooms. Although this made the job fun for me, I didn't keep it long. When there wasn't much to do, I was supposed to distribute crappy advertising flyers. I threw them in the trash and sat in a pub for three hours instead. The boss found that suboptimal and he fired me.

Fire at Will

2007. After a crisis year and a half of severe depression, I felt back on top of the world and decided to give my marriage and America another chance. Everything was unfinished. I couldn't come to terms with the fact that this chapter should be over already. My former work colleague Kerley from *Skypizza* offered me his help and I could stay on his couch for the time being until I found a job.

My parents didn't like the idea at all, they were worried. But they also knew that it was difficult to talk me out of something I had once set my mind to.

After I left again, a doctor said to my parents, completely bewildered, »How could you let him move to America alone in that condition?« It was also the time when stronger and stronger manic phases occurred, I was not aware of it. Mania is triggered by psychological pressure, or so my therapist says. With my second extended stay in the U.S., just on my own, I put myself under extreme pressure. I stopped taking my medication, I was doing well after all. Typical rookie mistake, please don't copy.

Kerley was kind enough to pick me up at Boston Logan International Airport. It felt great to be back in my second home and driving down the highway. I was ecstatic, another fresh start. Kerley was no longer working at *Skypizza* and was now working as a painter for 17 $ an hour, after all, at the pizza place it was only 8.25 $. He was from Brazil, always friendly, always laughing and only soccer on his mind. First we made a stop at his brother Werley's house. Kerley and Werley, what must their parents have been on. We sat down in the kitchen, drank some Budweiser, talked about old times and of course about soccer.

Say what you will about the Yanks, but every time I was over there, a little feeling of freedom filled me. That was certainly due to the size of the country, my expectations, nature and the easy-going feeling of the people there. In Germany, everything is a bit more regulated and conservative in everyday life, but the social freedom is much greater.

Many people think that Americans are shallow. That's partly true, but I can walk into a supermarket at 3:00 in the morning dressed only in a bathrobe, and completely bummed out pay for a can of Spaghetti and Meatballs for 65 cents with a check, they're always friendly at the register and smile at me. I'm sure they don't mean it seriously, but it makes me feel good and that's what it's all about.

Chicopee

Chicopee is the name of the small town just five miles from West-field. A little distance from Melonie seemed like a good idea; I didn't want to hassle her. I had 2,000 $ with me and gave myself a week to get settled. Most of the people living in the apartment complex were young people or young families. In the evenings, people they met at someone's house to chill out. I quickly enjoyed great popular-ity, I think it was because the Americans are not used to European openness. Of course, the reason could also have been that I always brought beer. Occasionally I sat with my new friends on the stairs in front of the house facing the street. I was manic and in an excessively overly cheerful.

One afternoon I went with them to a billiards parlor, we sat down at a table with guys who looked like gangsters: fat, black sugar daddies with gold chains and guns, a little scary. I felt like a foreign body and that's how they looked at me. A friend of mine wanted to play a game of betting pool and I idiot lent him 100 $. He lost and I never saw my money again. That was agreed, in retrospect I think they split the money. In general, in the USA it's always about the money. I remember how surprised I was when my wife paid Uncle Rob 20 $ for babysitting. I mean, within the family and even in the same house, it's natural to be helpful without asking for anything in return.

On Saturdays, Kerley's circle of friends got together to play soccer on a school field and I was proud as punch when I scored a goal against the Brazilians. I'm a really miserable player and the 7-1 at the 2014 World Cup hadn't happened yet. I called Melonie for the first time and told her about my sense of achievement. She was against me coming back to America, she hadn't processed it all yet, she told me. Contrary to my fear, she was in a good mood on the phone, then I remembered that it was Saturday and she was probably stoned in front of her computer.

In the evenings I cooked for Kerley's family mostly german classics like Schnitzel or cheese spaetzle and was able to make myself useful.

Coffestar

It was time to look for a job for myself. *Coffeestar* is always hiring, so I went in for an interview and the next day began my week-long training period. I moved in with Werley as a sublet, there was a *Coffeestar* store right across the street, just before the exit to the highway, early in the morning all hell broke loose. The rent for my small room was a whopping 400 $. I bought an air mattress. So I had a suitcase, an old laptop, for sentimental reasons a german flag, of course the air mattress and I was poor as a church mouse.

Early in the morning at 5:00 the alarm clock rang. An alarm clock, by the way, is something absolutely unnatural. My shift started at 6:00 a.m. and went until about 1:00 p.m., depending on how the preparations for the next day progressed. I quickly took on this additional task so that all employees could leave on time.

I always worked to the limit, memorizing all the regulars and what they ordered each day, so they didn't have to wait in line for long, I just waved them through. »This guy is amazing« and other positive reviews my boss often got to hear. At this point, however, I also have to mention that the employees' work morale was sub-par.

Many employees came to work kind of woozy, my buddy Joe was even on LSD occasionally.

They didn't care how many customers were in the store, they did their work in slow motion and probably didn't even know who or where they were. There was always something to laugh about, at least for me.

The mania got stronger, maybe you know when you are very exhausted and exhale loudly with a clearing of the throat. I was singing 'O sole mio' at opera volume in the morning at the store, dancing around and my brain was almost out of control, it was racing away so fast. More and more information I was storing unintentionally. After work, I went to the *P.N.O. Café* and other venues and entertained everyone present at the bar. Within four weeks I was known around town, everyone greeted me, even passing cars honked at me. I was bursting over with energy and it didn't go unnoticed. For example, a very old war veteran gave me a photo of him and his comrades, taken back in Nazi Germany, I restored it on the computer, he was pleased. I listened carefully in conversations, that is not a matter of course, at least not where I was now. With an insane speed and fullness I absorbed everything.

Melonie called me, she was going to Las Vegas for a party weekend hosted by our acquaintance Cathy and her husband Jimmy, and asked me for money. She wanted something from me, of course I agreed and the next day she actually came over, a reunion after a year and a half. I hugged her warmly and gave her a kiss on the cheek. She didn't like that very much and acted defensive. I gave her 200 $ and very cold she coolly said goodbye. Astonished, I thought to myself that true character is always revealed at or after a breakup. I was unsure if I could ever get her back. She was even angry with me because I had had the time in Berlin to have my depression treated in clinics.

Chicopee is a poor and fucked up small town, I realized. Everyone for himself and me for the most part. At the counter in the *P.N.O. Cafe*, one guy was paying and accidentally dropped two dollar bills, the two patrons to his left and right were fighting over them on the floor. I intervened and separated them. That's how low you can get, I was horrified. The amazing thing was: they both had jobs. That day, an older friend of mine named K.C. and I were drinking canned beer until dawn on some rooftop. I think I was still doing some kind of Native American dance until a tenant complained.

Beneath the superficially friendly society bubbled sheer survival instinct.

Over time, it dawned on me that America was sick and I was in the middle of it. The USA always seemed artificial to me, not real.

I met Yannik, he was from Poland and was stranded here. His mother was cleaning and he was unemployed. He took every drug that was available. It was summer and we would often go down to the river in the afternoons on a sneaky path through the woods, drink a few beers and talk, it was nice. Once we got some money left we would go to bars, unfortunately after a certain level Yannik would lose control and get into fights or get rowdy. I realized that he was no good for me and stopped seeing him.

Another constant was Alex, I called him 'Crazy' because he was constantly playing the same song again and again on the jukebox. An old, obnoxious guy who hung out exclusively in bars and licked his lips when he was too drunk and couldn't control his facial muscles. He was gay and had a crush on me. One night I attacked him and threw him across the room several times, he had gotten pushy before. He was lying on the floor with his cell phone in his hand and said to me, »You want me to call the cops? You're an immigrant, so piss off!« I had to admit defeat, I didn't want to get into trouble with the police.

400 $ rent a month was too much, a couple from the *P.N.O. Café* offered me a room for 200 $, they lived in the same building. Andy and Sue didn't have much money, shimmying from job to job, living hand to mouth. Good people in principle, who unfortunately got caught up in the drama of life. Like many in the place, they were occasionally on drugs, no, wrong - occasionally not on drugs. My room was about eight square meters, I had a black and white TV with a broken antenna and a musty bed. It was getting colder and never aired because heating costs were to be saved, windows were taped with foil. The whole apartment reeked of dust and cigarette smoke.

I took a second job at *Kick Off*, a sports bar with a kitchen. I was now the kitchen. It started at 3:00 p.m., and around 11:00 p.m. was closing time. Afterwards, I usually went to the *Turn Tavern*, a bar around the corner. Missy was the barmaid's name and she was hot as hell, a little too many tattoos, I'm not into that, but okay. If I had more to offer financially, my chances with her would have been greater. This sounds now as if I were a you're a fine friend, but Melonie was not there and behaved very dismissive.

Four hours of sleep and then another early shift at *Coffeestar*, life at the limit. Always this heavy exhaling, manic, revved up to the top. Slowing down was not possible. Meanwhile, times didn't matter at all, whenever I had time, I drank a few beers to switch off, just to have a brief moment to myself and relax. I often sat by the window at night and looked out, trying to realize where I was and what the hell I was doing here. I was in a very surreal movie. How I managed to do all that, I don't know, but it also led to me being so burnt out today. I needed all my strength and more.

I had done my second job well, the kitchen was back in the black, but still in a filthy condition. So I cleaned for two weeks, the boss was happy with the results. What was ridiculous was that all the restaurant chefs I met in the U.S. always stressed the need to protect their top-secret recipes. I had a hard time stifling a laugh, since it was always ready-made mixed together.

Reunion

I contacted Melonie, asked if I could come over, she said yes, Friday would be fine. We could go to *Froggies* for karaoke. Okay. I was very nervous, didn't want to make a bad impression, took the bus, a cab and arrived. My stepson Michael wasn't there and there was a new roommate, Wendy. Melonie often had roommates to help her pay the rent. No one lasted long with her, which confirmed my belief that it wasn't all me that had gone wrong. She needs people who admire her, even adore her, not everyone was willing to do that.

Anyway, Wendy was there - plus two guys I didn't know. We sat on the porch. I had hoped to be able to talk to her alone, after all, I had once again traveled halfway around the world to see her again. The atmosphere was extremely unpleasant, I felt unwanted and I decided to leave again. Shit happens. What had I done to make this woman so petrified of me? She had given me a Superman T-shirt when we first met. Apparently, I was supposed to save her. Apparently I didn't succeed.

She told me a few times that I lied to her. I think that is not true. Of course, I didn't tell her my negative qualities in detail, but I didn't lie.

Meanwhile, I can't stand women who lie on their backs like a bug and expect the man to do everything. Well, at least I got rid of my Hertha BSC jersey for Michael, I always brought one when I flew by. 'Michael' imprint and as a back number his respective age.

Months later, at Thanksgiving, I called Melonie again and asked her if I could possibly come over in the family circle. Since it is an important and traditional holiday in America, I had speculated on a yes. The family was happy to see me, Melonie was not. At the dinner table, I sat down next to her and she got up and took a seat elsewhere. I praised her mother for the delicious meal and Melonie's brother drove me back to Chicopee.

When I called my wife from work once, she was in a bad mood and called me names and a Nazi. That's probably the worst thing you can say to a German.

I preferred to spend Christmas with my old pizza buddy Brandon and his family, in the evening some of us went to play billiards at the *P.N.O. Café*. A nice evening, I was grateful, it did me good.

There was a woman who also occasionally frequented bars. Her son borrowed a few dollars from me from time to time. Even though I barely had anything myself, I didn't leave anyone out in the cold who had even less than I did. This woman was a little paranoid. She would sometimes yell »drug dealer« out of the blue, as if she were pressing a buzzer. She was referring to me, completely out of the blue. I really had nothing to do with such things. A dealer with a german accent would have been caught immediately. Not that I would have thought about it, I'm just saying.

Johnny was disabled, his running style was abnormal. I don't know what this disease is called, one leg always bends when running. In winter when it was slippery, he often fell down. I know it's not very nice, but that image in my mind always makes me giggle. We were good friends. He gave me a cross pendant from the Vatican that I wear to this day.

In a bar we sat together and watched baseball, the Red Sox played and won the championship. The Yanks call it the World Series, strange, it only takes place in America.

Without warning, tears suddenly shot out of my eyes, acute attack of depriviaton. That evening the staff found me on the floor by the toilets, I was depressed and had no strength left. I spent the night in a hospital. Johnny has become a priest, I was told, I hope he is well and I will see him again sometime.

Bavarian House

At *Kick Off* one evening, the chef from *Bavarian Haus* was present. A good two years before, Melonie and I had eaten there on the occasion of our wedding anniversary and, as the name suggests, they served German cuisine. He was called Jo and apart from me he was probably the only one in the village who came from Germany. I approached him and told him about my job situation and with a wink I brought in that it would be good to have someone authentic in his team. Two days later, this idea also sank into his cerebral cortex and we came to an agreement. I also got a free haircut so that I looked decent.

I quit *Coffeestar* and started working at *Bavarian Haus* for two dollars more an hour. The *Coffeestar* boss couldn't handle it all and told everyone that she had fired me.

It was a very large restaurant with a huge function room. About ten line cooks were always at work plus some kitchen helpers. Jo didn't know where to put me at first. I started something like a trainee program in the kitchen, later I was to become a host and look after the guests with my german accent.

At *Kick Off* I now had about three late shifts a week, and at *Bavarian House* six days. The stress remained at a very high level, but I got more money for my work.

By now it was October and there was a month-long Oktoberfest celebration in the large dining room, an huge logistical effort in terms of catering. The hall could fit about 300 guests, plus the people in regular service. I was in hardcore mode, functioning in cooking and as an entertainer. I was manic to the highest degree, animating people to sway, singing and explaining german customs, the guests were thrilled, the staff amazed.

Counted

On one day I was double booked, however, I could not be in two restaurants at the same time. Since Jo was paying more, I made a logical decision. The *Kick Off* fired me, the boss had an important family matter to care of that day and I was to run the place. He had not told me this beforehand and in retrospect I was very sorry and apologized several times, but could not reduce his annoyance with me.

There came the expected fireworks in my head and the big bang.

I sat on my bed and was completely burnt out and cried out of desperation, my head and body completely exhausted. In tears, I called the *Bavarian House* at night. Answering machine, I said I was pretty much fucked up and could not come to work tomorrow. The day after next I went back to work and still looked pretty destroyed. Jo just said with his back turned to me, »No show up, no job.« This fucker fired me for one fucking day of absence, claiming there was no message on the answering machine. He had used me for Oktoberfest, that's how I saw it. The employees were perplexed, too.

He gave me the last check and I went to the *Turn Tavern*, perplexed. Jacob, a waiter from the *Bavarian House*, was loitering at the counter, he was already over 60 and drank the frustration of his existence from his soul. I told him what had happened. He was also irritated, could not understand it, said that I had done everything right. He said that Jo was a tough boss and that he was also suffering, but at his age he was happy to have a job at all. In Germany, the *Bavarian House* wouldn't have survived even a month. At the risk of sounding like a bad thing, the food was no poster child for the german cuisine. The schnitzels were pounded to stamps and the breading was like glued on. The sausages produced in-house were not good, even the French onion soup was a joke. Salad dressings consisted of ready-made powder dumped together. Nevertheless, I always carried my little booklet in my shirt pocket and wrote down all the recipes. I once made the staff a proper Wiener Schnitzel, which Jo probably didn't like at all, understandably, because it made his kitchen look old, even if it was just a stinkin' normal Schnitzel. It was constantly drummed into you to always keep the same standards, consistancy, consistency. That makes sense, but being closed to new things can also be fatal for a gastronomic business. I always fell on deaf ears, all suggestions for improvement were shot down. I had a hard time with other alpha males in kitchens.

Town Pizza

The Turkish family that ran *Town Pizza* was very friendly. Mehmet had often seen me at *Coffeestar* in the morning, he noticed my eagerness to work. He asked me if I wouldn't like to work for him. Pizza maker was more my thing. I hadn't had a job for a week, which quickly becomes a problem in America, in no time you're sitting on the street. I said yes.

Six days a week for 13 hours each. The pay was 800 $ and I had to be available at all times, not a good deal. I told Mehmet about my landlords

Andy and Sue, their living habits and use of drugs. Without further ado he offered me to move in with him, a room and again a whopping 400 $ rent. I didn't get very far on the balance of 100 $ a week. It is common practice in the restaurant business to pay a fixed salary, but in return you have to work as much as the boss demands. It's no different in Berlin, hourly wages are avoided as much as possible. This is especially true with moonlighting. It's exploitation. And then these bosses also see themselves as great benefactors when they give you a pizza, a kebab or whatever for free. But they don't want to pay money.

At first, I didn't mind the long hours, but after a while I realized that this can't be a permanent state. Mehmet said to me, »Work hard for a better life.« That didn't make sense to me, what life?

The usual extended family design of immigrants in foreign countries looks something like this:

The whole family clan buys or rents a house together, where everyone lives. The money earned is collected in a pot and then occasionally a family member gets a car, for example. If someone gets a good job, the other family members are gradually brought into the company as well. In this way, a large family builds up its existence piece by piece. Quite clever, actually.

Working in traditional Turkish families is still a male thing, but since no one spoke fluent good english, Kelly was there to take the phone orders. Like me, she had already worked in the *Bavarian House*. She was still very young, maybe 20, and had no education to speak of; for example, she didn't know the difference between capitalism and communism. It was frightening, but she was a good soul, I liked her, even though she actually sat at the table all day and only raised her head when the phone rang.

One fine winter day she told me that Jo, the german boss of *Bavarian House*, had offered her a whopping 6,000 $ fucking dollars for a blowjob, salaried. She was fired, sued, and won in court. As it turned out, Jo was a really disgusting old German fuck.

My bipolarity eventually led to me being advised to look for another job. I broke down several times at work and could no longer handle the stress. I was allowed to continue working until I found new employment.

I recovered for a few days and went back to job hunting. I got an interview at *Fastfresh*, they couldn't believe I had been slaving away at the pizzeria for so little money. They offered me 10 $ an hour, gratefully I agreed. It was a fine little sandwich-and-burger joint, and all but Scott were very personable. Scott, unfortunately, was the chef, a pushy asshole and had about the level of a dead jellyfish. He talked incessantly. I assume he was on stimulants. He actually tried to explain to me how to cut a sandwich in half. We got into a fight a few times. I didn't have the strength to take the shit anymore, but kept going anyway. I still dream of seriously hurting him to this day.

In the meantime, just for a few days, I had an extra job in a restaurant outside, the boss was cool, an Irishman. I cut up buckets of chicken in a basement. My two colleagues were Russian and kept popping muscle relaxers to get by. That was now at the bottom and I quit.

Dani and the Blowjob

Mehmet and I moved to Schoolstreet, right next door was the *Raindogs*, a dark dive where mostly the unemployed frequented. There I met Dani, she was always very hyper and I quickly realized that she was manic-depressive like me. She was a math teacher and actually stood firmly in life. In her manic phases, she was at *Raindogs* from afternoons on and drank a lot, mostly Jägermeister shots with her beer. Jägermeister is very popular in the USA. We got along well and it didn't take long for us to become close. She had money and helped me out occasionally. She wrote on a piece of paper that she wanted to have children with me. She had fallen in love, I had not.

As we both stood outside another bar to smoke a cigarette, she pulled down my pants and gave me a blowjob, in broad daylight. People driving by bawled and honked their horns. Of course, word spread quickly in Chicopee, Scandal. I often went to the river with her, too, to enjoy a bit of nature and find peace. She confessed to me that she was married. I thought I wasn't hearing right.

Behind closed doors and windows, things are fierce in America.

Her husband now also came to *Raindogs*, oh man, he was about three times the size of me and a warehouse worker. He didn't know much, but Dani usually sat down next to me as a matter of course. I had a bit of a feeling she was provoking a confrontation between me and Goliath.

He said to me, »Hey man, let's go outside for a cigarette.« He had heard things, told me Dani was bipolar and he thought it would be good if I talked to her about her problems. At first I was relieved, he didn't know everything.

Like in every american bar, there were many TVs, I stared up at the right side, "Who wants to be a millionaire?" was on and I heard Goliath yelling at Dani and beating her up. I held back. Suddenly an anvil hit me in the back of my head, he went all the way, surprisingly I didn't get knocked out. Four people had to restrain him, he went berserk and even attacked a policeman in front of the door. In a rage he yelled at me: »I'm gonna kill my wife and then I will kill you!« I was a little stunned by the blow and sat still, had that really just happened?

Now I was really screwed, people started to be negative towards me, I had broken various small town rules. At work I accidentally cut my hand, it had to be stitched in the hospital, I was out for a week.

I hardly dared to go out on the street or into bars. I moved in with a friend for a week and went to the soup kitchen every day to get something to eat. The volunteers were surprised, I was the first and only one to thank them for the food. After that week I had no more options, I had to go back to Berlin, everything was going against me and I was just drawing on my last reserves. For two days I lived in the Boston airport, an employee at the information desk called me 'Sweetie' and she gave me five dollars. Completely devastated, I finally arrived in Berlin at the end of my tether.

End of Strength

In the period after America, my manic phases were more confused, at the peaks I even had mild delusions. I analyzed news intensively, paranoid I suspected conspiracies. I was of the opinion that I could virtually see through people. I felt everything incredibly strongly, I was no longer able to switch off. I'm not sure that I wasn't really able to see through people at that time. In mania, the brain is wide open and works fully automatically at full speed. At some point, the big bang occurs when it is no longer able to process all the information. It collapses as a protective measure. I like to compare this with the camera work from the Terminator's pont of view in the movie, everything is captured and evaluated at lightning speed.

Shortly before the end of the mania, at the peak, I get speech disorders. I am no longer able to pronounce my thoughts as quickly as they run through my head. The eyes twitch nervously in all directions.

In any hospital, psychiatric ward, or internal medicine department, there are always the »hello, help« callers.

They are very sick people, mostly very old and/or psychologically at the end of their rope. I feel infinitely sorry for them and realize where it all ends. Unless one is run over by a truck beforehand. That would be bad luck, of course. A normal, healthy person is not often confronted with this, but I am often in hospitals as a patient and see and feel all the misery. It scares me and I am not a doctor who knows how to deal with it objectively. My sister currently works as a doctor in an intensive care unit and I wouldn't want to trade places with her, it puts a lot of stress on her. Plus lots of overtime, two kids, half a zoo at home and no steady partner. Luckily our parents help her, without them it would not be possible.

My ex-US wife Melonie had separated from me in 2005. Before I returned to Berlin, I worked for about three months without even a day off, hanging out in bars. No time to breathe, plus way too spicy, greasy fast food. When I came back to myself in Berlin, I fell into the most severe depression ever and it lasted for years.

This brings us to my other 'all-time-favorite hospital' in Berlin-Zehlendorf, Internal Department.

I woke up one morning with incredible pain in my upper abdomen, off to the hospital. There it was determined that I had a severe pancreatitis. I had been living too unhealthily. I cried with pain and was transferred directly to the intensive care unit. A doctor I could recognize through my pain-distorted eyes said to me, »Only a leg amputation without anesthesia is worse.« I believed him immediately.

»On a scale of one to ten ... « ... »TWELVE, you dumb cow.«

It's like swallowing a bag of broken pieces, walking upright is barely possible. The pancreas is a nasty bitch, it doesn't recover. If you have such inflammations more often, you can practically count down the remaining years on earth, diabetes is to be expected. Inflammation is only bearable with morphine or opiates. The bitch acts as a distributor for all other organs, she is the light switch for everything, so to speak. If it's broken, it goes dark. An impertinence, I was pissed off. Obey, you fucking organ! When the doctor tells you, »This won't last much longer,« you realize that death can be very real and possibly very close. That didn't suit me at all, completely absurd that my life could be interrupted or even ended. I'm not finished yet, I haven't even finished yet.

For two weeks I was on a drip and was not allowed to eat, my body was flooded with intravenous fluids. I often crawled out of the four-bed room into the hallway, even to the nurses' station. I could take no more, the pain was so bad that I would rather die than have to endure it any longer.

I had never had a beer with Jeff Bridges, so I put off dying, there was no way I could disappoint the Dude.

My neighbor in bedmate had it worse. He was only 20 years old and had the same condition as me. Only a surgery could help him, the chance of him living longer was small. He was given three times as much Oxicodon as I was. He was only a skeleton now. Since we were both constantly drugged by the nurses, we got along great. His name was Thorsten and he had probably the ugliest plaid hat ever on his head. Despite exchanging contact information, I never heard from him again. I guess he didn't make it.

I now have to watch what I eat and drink. I did not understand the cause of this disease at first. I mean, of course I have always lived very wildly, but compared to others I have moved rather mediocre. These health problems are eating away at my psyche and when I am manic, I have no control over myself and usually end up in the hospital for at least a week. That saps my strength. Once I even had 800 milliliters of water in my lungs. It usually hurts a lot when they stick a cannula through your back to suck out the fluid. I'm so used to all that, I don't even flinch anymore, at most with an eyebrow.

Her name was Alfreda, Norbertine or Krimhild, she always sat outside in the smoking corner in her wheelchair. Her leg had been amputated and she had a stent in her chest. Physically, she must have been about 140 years old, but she was only a little over 60 and smoked easily three packs of cigarettes a day. Sitting there, she was bitter and vicious. She virtually nagged with her spent voice (Even Tom Waits would be jealous.). As soon as the fat sister, Tina, appeared, she started to bitch about her. It would be unhealthy to be so fat, tirades of insults followed. After half a week my patience and the thread tore and I told her very clearly my opinion, I took her with only a few sentences humanly and psychologically completely apart. It was mean, but she deserved it. It's not a good idea to tease me. From then on she was overly kind to me, which surprised me.

Pancreatic inflammation usually also has something to do with excessive alcohol consumption. We were always a party-loving family. Sports and partying, that's how I grew up. My childhood in the 70s and 80s was characterized by out-of-home and social-partying habits. As a teenager, around the age of 14, I was consequently always in the front row when someone shouted »Paaaarty!«. From an early age, I was taught that people rewarded themselves for achievements with alcohol and generally functioned better in society. People are then always more cheerful.

However, if psychological problems are added to this, as in my case, it can lead to alcohol abuse in terms of coping with problems. The effect of alcohol is known to be different for each person, I become more happier, creative and feel more confident. Conversely, that means I'm usually more insecure, that's true.

In depressive phases I hardly drank anything, in mania almost uncontrollably. I always kept my hands off the hard alcohol. I would describe myself as a social alcoholic, at home there's water, but out there I feel better with a beer, then I can put on my show. I let my emotions run wild and feel more alive.

These days, I hardly drink at all. My doctor says I have to give up my slovenly lifestyle. I've also stopped smoking. All well and good, but it's boring. I have to try to find something positive in life without partying, not so easy if you're me.

Back then, after my return from America, I tried to settle back in Berlin. I often went to the *Grillhaus*, a kebab shop. At the counter, I made plans to open a pizzeria. The turkish boss smelled a rat and asked me if I wanted to make pizza at his place. He was an immigrant who had actually walked from Turkey to Germany. Respect. He is a peasant, very simple-minded and stuck with age-old values. For him, only money counts, nothing else. He regularly beat his girlfriend from Poland in the back room of the kebab store and she drank a lot of vodka to endure it.

I thought, okay, why not? I started to get the oven, pizza plates, sliders and all the other stuff, the making line had to be rebuilt, my very handy father helped. After a few tests I managed to make a very good pizza, a mix of american and italian recipes. You wouldn't think it, but pizza is a science in itself. Cooking has become one of my favorite hobbies over time.

Since Iwas solely responsible for the pizza, I always had to be present, 13 hours a day, every day of the week. I was paid a salary of 750 euros. After five months without a break and extreme mania, I quit, I couldn't take it anymore. I got out of control and ended up in a psychiatric ward again. Sometimes I still dream of having my own restaurant, but it also fulfills me to cook for the family once a week, that's enough for me.

Psychiatry

In a psychiatric ward, all the windows are always locked, you can guess why. Slowly, figures creep through the hallways, staring aimlessly with empty eyes. The medication handouts and feedings are the highlights of the day. In daily group rounds, patients sit in a circle of chairs and one by one are asked how they are doing and if they slept well. Group therapies are usually the order of the day in a loony bin. Activation group, depression group, addiction group, occupational therapy, some kind of memory training, and much more.

I have been to such a facility about 15 times so far. I have no choice but to go there when I can no longer control my thoughts and myself. Then I need some help and rest to come back to myself. Most of the time I am brought down with medication first. The therapies that are offered there are always the same and don't help me. They may work for other patients, of course. Occupational therapy is an exception, I can be creative and paint or do crafts, I find that relaxing and it brings me back a bit to the person I actually am.

Paradoxically, they give me strong psycho pills at night, which sedate me and make me very sleepy. At the same time, they expect me to be on the mat early in the morning at 7:30 a.m. and participate in exercise therapy before breakfast, preferably with an ice bath. With this, they try to physically fight the depression. It doesn't help with me. My play instinct gives me some lift. Whenever there is a ball in sports, I can't help it, I have to chase it. That's fun for me.

It often happens that a therapy leader is just 21 years old and wants to teach me something about life. All I can do is smile wryly. Of course, the next generation has to start somewhere, but please do it with someone who has experience. Savings are completely out of place at this point.

There are only a few drugs that are used in psychiatric wards, with them being dosed back and forth. Certainly, it plays a role which pharmaceutical company is behind it and how much money can be earned or saved with it. There are quite a few reports, investigations and conspiracy theories circulating on the Internet. My therapist told me the other day that they were now even using MDMA and ketamine for depression. But I don't want to get into that for now, that's not what this is about.

It's about jam. I hate orange or apricot marmalade and no matter how often I tell them in the clinic or even write it down, I always get red marmalade once and orange marmalade once for breakfast. And this jam, not wanted by all the patients, piles up in the refrigerators until it eventually has to be disposed of. Get one thing straight:

Nobody wants orange jam!!!

(except the island apes)

Often the patients are first immobilized, for me mostly too calm, emotionally switched off. The visits by the doctors are far too short, uncharitable and superficial. In principle, it is only a matter of being adjusted to the medication. Depressed people in particular are usually destroyed souls who are trying to pick themselves up again. The alternative is suicide, because hanging on is a difficult war with oneself in the long run, self-confidence is almost non-existent. Some of my friends lost this battle and took their own lives. My view of things has changed a lot, whether that's a good thing I don't know yet. Freedom and carefreeness are mostly gone, gratitude became stronger.

How many times did I have to hear: »Heeey, everybody sucks sometimes.« This lack of understanding annoys me. But they can't know any better, they don't have a clue about how severe this disease is, how much it limits life and how threatening it is.

It is a very personal disease that wreaks havoc deep in the soul.

It happened that my sister recognized manic states and admitted me to the psychiatric ward. They were very extreme states of mind. In a Brandenburg clinic, I was strapped down in an observation room for two days, that's how violent I was. I screamed and cried. It was a terrible place, the nurses were cold and unfriendly, kind of like the ward manager in the movie *One Flew Over the Cuckoo's Nest*. Just about everything was forbidden. I was not allowed to leave the institution and my laptop was retained. At 10:00 p.m. they checked if the lights were off in the rooms. If I wanted to smoke a cigarette, I had to get permission first. There was a fenced garden area where inmates were allowed to be for a few hours a day. It was like being in a cage. It was a drug-soaked nonentity; the patients were just kept. I was put on an anti-epileptic drug, for three months I lived completely emotionless, then I stopped it, it wasn't me anymore.

For two years, so-called counselors came to visit me once a week. The conversations usually ended with them leaving completely disillusioned. Caregivers and cared-for people met monthly to go bowling. My fellow sufferers were not particularly interesting, but I liked to bowl, even if not well.

Since my last longer stay in hospital, I was now taking a medication with a Q at the beginning of its name in a very high dose. It made me a little slow in the head or just normal, if you will. The fact that I was prescribed Q was to take its revenge.

During a therapy session, my couchologist looked up Q. There is a warning in the 'Red List' (special book for doctors about side effects of medications) because the drug can cause pancreatitis. Excuse me? Whaaat?

In the psychiatric ward, despite a known pancreatic sensitivity, they had prescribed me a drug that can cause pancreatitis. And I wondered why I kept ending up in the hospital. What I went through all those years, the pain, the fear of death, and likewise the psychological impact. I was stunned.

My organ has sustained significant damage that will never go away. My life expectancy has decreased significantly, I will get diabetes. These assholes did this to me, I have never been so angry in my life. Very big fuck you finger.

If you are also affected and have been prescribed a medication that starts with a Q, check it out very carefully. Check the 'Red List' and dose it down slowly in consultation with your doctor. Look around for alternatives. I can't mention the name of the drug, they would sue me right immediately.

And now to something completely different:

I had read on the Internet that there are so-called affiliate casino earning opportunities. It works like this: I design a website with information, for example, about roulette systems and strategies. The visitor to my website clicks on the advertisements of online casinos that I have placed and if the person gambles away, let's say 100 euros in these casinos, I get half of his losses. At that time, I was taking only antidepressants, that is, no medication to prevent me from mania, and I worked every day for 16 hours like a man possessed. After a year, I had six extensive websites online. These days I'm not as work-aholic, and I'm sure that's partly due to the pills I have to take. A common side effect is listlessness.

For a few years I lived in my parents' basement. I was not well. I was severely depressed. Of course, it was very kind of them to let me stay there, but I felt inferior and was looking for independence and more distance from the family. I don't even remember how it came about, but one evening I ended up at the *Roxy Café* in Teltow, a run-down dive. The beer didn't cost much, and I went there often. The mania also made an occasional appearance, I danced completely unleashed from time to time and the many people ballasted me in conversation with their problems.

Too much information, I went on another flashy mental glary-thought-carousel.

A primitive audience, I don't like to say that, but that's the way it was. Although I was quickly popular because of my social nature and because I could listen , just as quickly I had enemies who didn't like my leather clothes and long hair. Many people were politically to the far right. One girl noticed that my facial expression was always sad, she said that to me. One guy chatted me up, he had heared that I was good with computers. His plan was that he would steal cars and I would be in charge of the software and disguising its origin. He was about the most antisocial ass I'd ever met and he was always stinking drunk. I declined the offer without thanks.

I had a new scooter and parked behind the store. My rear view mirrors were stolen and I could guess who it was. I was summoned by the police a few weeks later to testify. I told what I knew and refrained from pressing charges, since there were no witnesses. Problem: The prosecutor had known the guy for some time and decided to press charges despite the lack of evidence. When I showed up at the *Roxy Café* again, I was beaten up by this pisser. I lost my upper front teeth and had to pay a whopping 800 € for two new ones.

Some people at the *Roxy* wore sweaters or T-shirts that said, 'No mercy for child molesters.' Nobody in the world, except the church, would ever demand mercy for child molesters. It's just a psycho trick of Nazis to recruit new members for the respective party with simple statements. So bad cheap, but stupid people fall for it.

Since 2013 I live alone in a nice one-room apartment in Kleinmachnow, I do not need more. There is not much in Kleinmachnow, rich Westerners moved here after the reunification, it is a beautiful suburb of Berlin. I would love to move back to Berlin-Zehlendorf, where I grew up, but it's just too expensive for me. Because of the manic-depressive illness, I get a lousy pension for reduced earning capacity. I have to live below the poverty line.

I still wanted to do the some economic studies over two years, but the long way there by public transport was psychologically a torture for me, shortly before graduation and after another stay in a psychiatric clinic I did not go there again.

In the meantime, I've been volunteering to help refugees. And while we're at it:

You stupid, antisocial right-wing rage citizens can kiss my ass.

Sorry, that had to come out now.

For about four years now I've been limiting part of my social life to a kebab store, I can still afford that, most of the time anyway. In summer I'm at the Schlachtensee lake and meet some friends. The six months of fall and winter, on the other hand, are very lonely. It makes me sad and I can't think of a way out. Most of the time I write in the kebab store or listen to music. The regulars in the snack bar tend to be of a simpler disposition, window and door makers, bus drivers, the unemployed, but also some pensioners looking for social support.

The owner and his employees are Kurds, we often discuss Erdogan's anti-democratic policies. A very nice employee is called Bahoz Yildirim, I promised to mention him in this book. Kind regards.

Hermann and Julius are both over 70 years old and regulars. Hermann chats at length every day without a period about the weather and Julius talks constantly about young, handy women, fucking and Viagra. And then there is Karl, 60 years old, drinks a lot, is addicted to gambling and talks to himself when he is drunk and rants about God and the world. He is a minibus driver for children and disabled people. Whenever he has too much booze with his beer, he gets loud and aggressive. Most of the time he is in debt to the Kurdish boss of the store and the other day he actually yelled »Foreigners out!« in his state. He had to listen to a lot from me, I don't keep quiet. The other day Karl said, »I have teletext, I don't need a newspaper.« Brilliant moments that I enjoy very much.

What a crappy year. I'm currently sitting in a restaurant where I was still employed as a pizza maker in 2008, the ad is still visible outside as a neon sign. Yesterday at noon I was released from the hospital.

At the end of November, I was taken the right of way, my scooter is scrap and I was for a week with a brain hemorrhage in a Potsdam hospital. After that, I wasn't really in a good mood, completely off track, and then over Christmas my pancreas gave me pain, hospital again, no Christmas Eve with the family. The ultrasound doctor said to me, »I'm sorry, Mr. Brodeur, you're still so young.« That sentence blew my mind. I get opiates as a short infusion in the clinic. That's the only way to bear the pain. Later, it gets funny when I'm not in pain anymore and the stuff is still in the patient schedule. When the nurse leaves the room, I turn up the infusion full blast and I'm really fine for half an hour. Less funny was an older gentleman who was placed next to me in the room and smelled like shit, I slept next to him for a week.

I wonder why I didn't die when I was 27. It's rock n' roll, that's how I've been ever since I can remember, and now I have to be different, grown up and sensible. I just can't.

I wished Lotta a happy new year despite her no contact policy and she even replied. I think a lot about the past and where I am now. I am often worried. Is this it already? Is there nothing more to come now? Will it stay this way and what can I do about it? Although I expect it from my therapist, she rarely gives me practical and useful advice.

On New Year's Day, I was exhausted, also psychologically, and called a few clinics; there were no beds available. I needed time to process and to think. Finally, in Potsdam, an institution that I know from my own experience and don't like had a place free, of necessity I agreed and the next morning I checked in there. However, the place was free in the addiction ward and not in the psychiatric ward. I didn't care at that moment.

After just over a week I was discharged again, I was not an addiction patient, they reasoned. Of course, compared to the other inmates, I probably wasn't. There were new admissions with four parts per thousand and the next day these poor saps sometimes had really severe withdrawal symptoms and had to be treated with medication. There were guys who had been there twenty times and tried again and again to get the addiction problem under control, in vain. But I think it's a sign of strength to keep trying. Respect. There was a slimmed-down version of the usual therapy offerings in the mental health department, and the detoxification of the patients was the main focus here.

The first two days I didn't say much, I was paralyzed by the previous events, sitting in a sofa corner in the lounge and indulging in my favorite pastime: Observing. Some loudmouths were setting the tone and were constantly agitating against foreigners. I am shocked at the extent of the now blatant way of establishing radical right-wing ideas as normal. From 7:00 p.m. the TV was allowed to be turned on and it was decided to watch a Hitler documentary, fuck. I was very tired and went to sleep. I thought about how to avoid falling into such deep abysses in the future, which cause these damaging inflammations. Also, I don't want to be such a burden to my parents with my problems anymore. I wrote down some resolutions and dos and don'ts that I should stick to.

A therapist noticed my crucifix pendant and said to me, »You are smarter than God, he keeps shooting lightning bolts at you and you always manage to dodge.« She was probably trying to tell me that this can't go on forever.

Some of the right-wing antisocials were released and the stay became more comfortable. A small, relatively soft community formed and we talked openly about our problems. I got a few hugs goodbye. Even the kitchen fairy told me when I left that I had been a very nice patient. Peace and diplomacy – I`m good at.

At the beginning of the book, I said that bipolarity is usually accompanied by excessive aids as well. It is a very fine line on which one tries to balance oneself. I wish everyone affected strength and luck in this.

Fade-Out

Melonie now only contacts me when she wants something from me, such as my Social Security number for taxes or cooking recipes. She has stopped contacting me on social media, as has Lotta. Both did it after I informed them that I was writing a book.

While I see the beautiful moments in the relationships, they would prefer not to be reminded of them. I suppose they just want to move on with their lives detached from the past. I understand the discomfort when someone writes something about you, and I hope I've been fair about it.

I have always been a somewhat destructive person, I can't make anyone happy with that, I realize. The other day, a pal wrote to me via Facebook, saying she would like to meet me again to talk. I know her from the psychiatric ward. I have determined for myself not to have any special contact with people I have met in clinics. An old love, with whom I am also still in contact, wrote to me that I would always do magic. What she meant by that, I don't know. I hope I don't seem too arrogant, but it must also be allowed to stand by one's own strengths, that is healthy for the psyche. I also talk openly about my many weaknesses.

After all the strength-sapping hospital stays, attempts at medication, illnesses, pain and changing life circumstances, I find it difficult to internalize a consistent image of myself. I am unsettled, but at the same time I see and feel everything frighteningly clearly and completely.

How many times have I tried to explain to my girlfriends and my wife that I am in fact someone else. How many times did I have to apologize for things I normally would never have said or done. So often I was confused and floundering helplessly, so often I was desperate and didn't know what to do.

I feel like I've missed ten years. All of a sudden I'm 46 years old, living in a one-room apartment again, a hairdresser recently trimmed my ear hair without being asked, and the commercials assures me that there's no more plutonium in my shampoo. I still have minimal social contacts, but I wouldn't tolerate more. I'll be glad when people leave me alone after the big storm. Right now I don't want to put myself out to any woman, the poor thing would be completely overwhelmed and I would probably make someone miserable again.

The outlook for the rest of my life is unclear. I hope I will become healthier again; at least physically. I am trying. It would be unpleasant if my circumstances remained like this forever. I believe that I will succeed in making a new start. I am far from finished, I have just begun. I will try to bring out again the person I once was, the one who was buried under all this. I have gone all the way in life, I don't regret that, other people would need three lifetimes for that.

In therapy, we occasionally read my texts together. My therapist noticed that I always write positively. That surprised me; I had never perceived myself as a positive person.

What really pisses me off is that after I die, everything just goes on and I can't be there. I had always wished to be everywhere in the world at the same time. I experienced this feeling, a gigantic feeling, I don't even remember when and where I had it. Was I on drugs, was I having sex, or was it during a near-death experience?

You're probably thinking I'm nuts now. I don't deny that, I can't change it, like so many things in life. I take myself as given and make the best of it. You should do the same, this way you can better deal with yourself and the world. Accept yourself with all your strengths and weaknesses, do things that do you good, surround yourself with friends, love your family and always have a treat for the dog.

On that note, thank you for your attention. I hope you enjoyed the book.